The Busy Woman's Guide
to
Inner Health
and
Outer Beauty

Meredith Yardley

www.meredithyardley.com

Disclaimer

Although the author and publisher have made every effort to ensure that the information in this book was correct at time of print, the author and publisher do not assume and hereby disclaim any liability to any party for any loss, damage, or disruption caused by errors or omissions, whether such errors or omissions result from negligence, accident, or any other cause.

This book is not intended as a substitute for professional medical advice. The reader should consult a medical practitioner in matters relating to his/her health and particularly with respect to any symptoms that may require diagnosis or medical attention.

In this book I offer a number of suggestions to the reader for goods and services. I may receive a commission or affiliate payment for some of these. I only suggest goods and services I have used myself and am 100% happy with.

* * *

MEREDIAN
PICTURES & WORDS

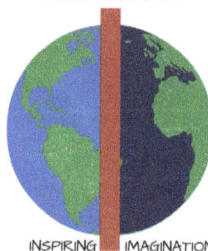

INSPIRING   IMAGINATION

Foreword
by Michelle Duffield

Being a professional endurance triathlete is not a usual career. It requires determination. It requires commitment. It requires training and competing, even when it's the last thing I feel like doing.

But in some ways, my job may be much like yours. There is a lot of pressure in my chosen field. If you work in the corporate world, or run your own business, or have a high pressure job of any sort - you'll know what I mean.

There are two types of pressures - the pressure people put on us, and the pressure we put on ourselves. I think the pressure we put on ourselves to succeed, particularly in a masculine-dominated world (for me it's sport, for you it might be law, or engineering, or finance or medicine), can be far more intense than the pressure other people put on us.

I am learning that sometimes I will rise to my own expectations, and other times I need to forgive myself when I try, but fall short. Maybe it's like that for you too.

For me, my journey through sport has taught me a few lessons that have stood by me and helped me get to where I am now. I found that these lessons are very much aligned with the messages in Meredith's book.

When it comes to health and wellbeing I have three guiding principles:

1   Dream so big it's scary.
2   Daily habits are where it's at.
3   You may fall. Accept and move on.

Dream so big, it's scary. If your dreams don't scare you, they aren't big enough. As humans we are creatures of habit and often fear the unknown - but it is outside the limits of our experiences and achievements that the greatest gains are to be had. This is where life begins. The scarier it is, the greater the sense of accomplishment when you achieve it.

Dream about who you want to be and what you want to achieve tomorrow, next year, even five years from now. Life is precious, and it will pass you by. When your time is up, what do you want others to say about you? Will you be one of those old ladies who jumps out of an airplane to celebrate their 85th birthday? (Well, you may not want to, but don't you want to be healthy enough that you have the choice?) Perhaps you want to be a healthy role model not just for your kids (or nieces, nephews, other people's kids - you get the idea), but also your friends, family and even colleagues. Whatever you would like to be, make a start on it. Today.

Daily habits are where it's at. Meredith devotes a quite a bit of time looking at a number of ways people can install new habits. We're all different, so different things will work for different people and this may take a bit of trial and error before you decide what works for you.

It is so true that 'from little things, big things grow'. This applies to the seemingly insignificant habits we do each and every day. While individually they may seem harmless and of little consequence, they add up when continued frequently over a longer period of time. Eventually the compound effect kicks in and BOOM, your little daily habit has a dramatic impact on your life.

So it's vital that your daily habits are ones that will support you in the direction you want to go. After all, daily habits have got you to where you are now, haven't they? Small and frequent deposits into your habit routine will eventually see you achieve your goals. Your habits can hinder you - or help you. You make the choice.

Know your habits, and don't feel guilty about the occasional treat. Know it's just a treat, not part of your usual routine and just enjoy it for what it is.

You may fall. Accept and move on. We are human beings. Not perfect, not robots, and Meredith is very clear about the need to be realistic and pragmatic about yourself and your expectations. She gives you information, and ideas, about how you might incorporate new ways of being into your life.

Take nutrition for example. Meredith gives you information about what types of foods can assist you in being healthy, and what will not serve you. Then she gives some practical examples of what you can do to incorporate these ideas into your life. Some are just one or two tweaks, some are bigger shifts. She provides checklists (because she knows you're super busy like me) that can really help when you just need a quick reminder and don't have time to read a whole chapter.

You will always face challenges, barriers and obstacles that make your journey difficult. If you choose to learn from your setbacks, take another tack and keep going, you will have a pretty good chance of getting where you want to be. For me, one my career highlights came as a result of one of my worst performances.

Rather than achieving my expectation in my first attempt at the Ironman World Championships in Hawaii - I fell well short of my goal. It was a tough pill to swallow. But when I reviewed the race, my approach and preparation, I was able to identify what to do differently next time.

In 2013 I returned to that race a different athlete. I had applied the lessons I learnt from my first attempt, and returned with a new sense of confidence that I had become the athlete I needed to be, to get the results I knew I could get. That year I finished second in my age group, and 33rd female overall. I really believe that without that 'fall' in 2011, I would not have learnt the lessons necessary to return two years later to achieve the second result. It was my results in 2013 that set me on my professional athletic path. Without that experience, and what I learned from it, I could never have achieved what I have since.

Having worked in the corporate world, spending month after month living in and out of suitcases and in hotel rooms - Meredith knows sometimes things just have to be taken one step at a time. So it's okay to fall, to slip, to drop into old habits. Just recognise them for what they really are - a small step in your learning to be a healthier you.

Meredith's message of not being too hard on yourself, and allowing yourself to learn and grow is key to making the changes you want to achieve your goals. And isn't that what we all want - to live a healthier, more fulfilling life? I know I do, and since you're reading this book, you probably do too.

Michelle Duffield

You can keep up to date with Michelle via Instagram @mimduffield and her website www.michelleduffield.com.

Want a Bonus Chapter for FREE?

As a thank you for ordering a copy of my book, I'd like to give you a Bonus Chapter for free!

Is Your Skin Care a Health Hazard? has a look at many of the chemicals that manufacturers put in personal care products. The best way for you to choose high quality personal care products is to know what's in them, and what that means for your skin and your health. That way, you can make informed decisions about what you buy. I want you to choose well.

To get your copy, just email me at meredith@meredithyardley.com and I'll send it right to you!

Contents

Introduction

I don't know about you - but one day I woke up, looked in the mirror and, without any warning, I just looked older.

And I thought about all those women who look so elegant, who seem to age so beautifully. Women in their 40s, 50s and 60s and older, looking fabulous. Women like Catherine Deneuve, Sophia Loren, Michelle Pfeiffer, Glenn Close and Helen Mirren.

I want to be one of them. Don't you?

I'm not afraid of ageing, but that day I saw myself looking older I wondered 'Has my chance passed me by? Have I left it too late to age gracefully? What would I tell my younger self so I can look gorgeous as I get older, so I can age gracefully?'

So I decided to do some research. To my relief, I found out that no, I have NOT left it too late. I can start taking care of my skin at any age. And if I do it properly, not only will I put off looking old, I can actually nourish myself through my skin at the same time.

What I found out was just so simple, so easy, so commonsensical (is that a word?) I wondered why I hadn't already done it.

And then I thought, 'It's not just me who can do this. There are millions of women who have the same thoughts that I do when they look in the mirror every day'.

So I wrote this short book. Short because I know you have lots of demands on your time. Short so you can easily dip in and out of it at any time. And because I want to make things even easier for you, I have included some little gems that you can access through the very pages of this book.

Gems such as:

- A checklist of what to look for in your skin products to make sure you are getting a value product with quality ingredients.
- A little video you can access through my book that shows you exactly how to follow a beauty routine that is quick, easy and full of nourishing goodness.
- A list of Skin Superfoods explaining the things you can eat that will help plump up those little skin cells to reduce obvious wrinkles.
- A list of questions to ask yourself (and the manufacturer) of the skin care products you choose to make sure it really is the best quality product for your health.
- And yes, I'm going to talk about guts and poop - because no-one ever tells you these things and yet they are CRITICAL to your continued good health.

So get reading. If you have any queries, just follow the links to my blog (meredithyardley.com), email me at meredith@ meredithyardley.com, or connect with my Facebook page at www. facebook.com/enrichingyourenergy.com.

BLOG

E-MAIL

FACEBOOK

Oh, make sure you grab your copy of the Bonus chapter called 'Is Your Skin Care A Health Hazard?'. In it I look at the chemicals added to many personal care products and ask what are they, ask are they really necessary, and I explore what they can do to you.

I'd love to hear from you – questions, comments, even suggestions for my next book – all are welcome. Just send me an email at meredith@meredithyardley.com.

My mission is to help all of us care for and love the skin we live in. And even more, to love and care for ourselves.

Cheers!

Meredith

Chapter 1
Is your gut making you ugly?

*'People often say that beauty is in the eye of the beholder.
I say that the most liberating thing about beauty is
realising that YOU are the beholder.' - Salma Hayek*

Don't we all want to feel beautiful?

I know I do. I'm not so much worried about looking like a fabulous model in a magazine, or a film star behind a soft lens. But I want to **feel** beautiful - have clear, healthy skin, walk with confidence, and be proud of my laugh lines.

A desire to age gracefully sent me on the journey that has become this book - and I have discovered some amazing things. I hope you enjoy reading about them as much as my research has been fun for me.

How the health of your gut is reflected in your face

The quality of your skin will be determined by what goes on in the inside of your body more than what you do on the outside.

Poor digestion or an unbalanced gut can reflect in your skin. There are many reasons for poor digestion or gut problems. Some are serious conditions needing a diagnosis, such as coeliac disease, ulcerative colitis and Crohn's Disease.

However I'm not going to discuss anything like that here, as these conditions need medical assistance. If you think you are suffering from any of them, see your doctor or health professional as soon as you can. I just want to share with you what I've found out about good digestive health.

There is a reason I'm pretty keen on you treating your gut with love.

I started to suffer from bloating when I reached my mid-40s. I could not believe how uncomfortable, and sometimes how painful, it could be.

So I trotted along to a gastro specialist for the top and tail (endoscopy and colonoscopy) to get checked out for anything nasty.

There was good news. There was bad news. The good news was there was nothing to find, not even a polyp.

The bad news was that they couldn't tell me what was wrong. 'Medically diagnosed irritable bowel syndrome' was the only answer I got, but no suggestions on how to rid myself of it or even how to manage it.

It obviously was not very helpful. So I figured I would have to do my own research. I want to share this with you because I don't want you to suffer for as long as I did before getting some answers, and some relief. And even if you don't suffer from bloating, cramping and general digestive upsettedness, what I discovered is, in fact, just a good digestive health recipe to follow which everyone should know about.

Your Gut – The Home of Your Body's Immune System

Where do you think your immune system is based? Bet you didn't think it was in your gut. But wonder of wonders, it is.

In fact, there is even evidence that after taking gut microbes from a healthy rat and implanting them into an unhealthy rat, the unhealthy rat got better.

Even more weird, as reported in 2010 in several publications including *New Scientist*, a woman who was dying of bowel cancer was given a faeces transplant. Before you say 'eeeuuuhhh, too disgusting', **this treatment saved her life**. This woman was close to death. She had lost 27 kilos and was suffering from almost fatal diarrhoea (every 15 minutes). Nothing the doctors did was successful. Within two days of the fecal transplant, she had gone from diarrhoea to solid bowel movements, and she continued to improve, ultimately recovering entirely.

I'm not telling you this to gross you out. I'm telling you this to give you an example of how amazing your gut is. So you really understand that the health of your gut is central to the health of your entire body and mind.

Your Gut - Your Body's Second Brain

In 400 BC, Hippocrates, the father of modern medicine, wrote '*Death sits in the bowels*' and '*Bad digestion is the root of all evil*'. Hippocrates knew his stuff.

Our gut is full of bacteria. Before you say 'EEEWWW!' know that this is a Good Thing. Well mostly. There are bad bacteria in your gut too. But let's focus on the good bacteria first. Numbering about one hundred trillion bacteria, there are more microbes in your gut than there are stars in the Milky Way! It is the most dynamic ecosystem on our planet. The health of these microbes affects everything in your body from immunity to mental health.

And the best news is I found the solution to my cramping and bloating was simple - and, even better, inexpensive. Probiotic - hard working little soldiers

I regularly take a good quality probiotic as it helps balance the flora in my gut. Keeping your gut healthy will make a huge difference, not only to the quality of your skin, but to the quality of your life.

Antibiotics are wonder drugs, there is no doubt about it, but they do have a downside. And that is that antibiotics kill off good bacteria as well as bad bacteria. So the good bacteria need to be supported to grow and multiply.

If you are taking antibiotics, wait an hour or so then take your probiotic. This will help support the good gut bacteria that, unfortunately, your antibiotics will have reduced in their search and destroy mission for the nasties that are making you ill.

Many studies have shown probiotics have significant health benefits, including improved immune function (because your immune system is based in your gut); protection against bad bacteria and possible infection; improved digestion and absorption of food.

It is also suggested that probiotics can help break down protein and fat - which is great for anyone with a compromised digestive system.

Even if you don't feel your digestive system is compromised, it is widely believed in the integrative health field that taking a regular probiotic is beneficial for your gut.

Prebiotic inulin - food source for the goodness in your gut

So you've heard about the benefits of probiotic, but I bet you haven't heard of a PRE-biotic called inulin.

What exactly is inulin and why is it good for our digestive system?

Inulin (not insulin which regulates your blood sugar) is colourless and tasteless. It is present in the chicory root from which it's extracted (the root of green leaf witlof. It's also in other vegetables and some grains in small amounts such as Jerusalem artichoke.)

It's a starchy carbohydrate - read fibre - that our bodies can't digest. It feeds the 'friendly' bacteria that live in our large intestine. These bacteria break down the inulin and feed off it, they grow and blossom and this contributes to a healthy digestive system.

Inulin is also a fibre that enhances the soluble fibre in other foods stuffs we ingest (soluble fibre is fibre that can be broken down by your digestion). It adds bulk to your food (helping reduce your kilojoule intake) and helps lower blood cholesterol. However it's not a 'whole food' like brown rice or legumes so you wouldn't want to count on inulin as your only fibre content.

Inulin is used in drinks, bars, yoghurts and powders to add a creaminess and boost the bulk of the product. I use it in powder form as an addition to my morning protein shake, or sprinkled on my quinoa porridge or fruit salad.

Just as an aside, I have chosen the products I use for very specific reasons. They are manufactured to pharmaceutical standards, not just food standards. They are used by over 1000 elite and professional athletes, around the world. The company holds itself to the highest manufacturing standards, opening itself up to independent auditing several times a year. If you'd like to know more, email me at meredith@meredithyardley.com or check out what I use at www.enrichyourenergy.usana.com. Fibre - keeps you moving.

EMAIL

WHAT I USE

Keeping your gut moving is what it's all about. Unless you eat lots of vegetables and fruit (seven different types, five times a day), some whole grains, cultured milk products, and fermented products like sauerkraut, your insides will probably need a bit of help.

It's amazing what will sit in your large intestine for a long time. I have even heard of a middle-aged man who had a colonic and a small plastic toy he swallowed when he was a child floated down the tube. It took a few colonics for this to dislodge, but it's an indication of how long something can sit in your gut.

A good quality fibre additive can work wonders, especially if it's a powder and you can hide it in your food such as egg dishes or baking, smoothies or shakes. Make sure you drink a lot of liquid (and I don't mean wine or vodka!) when taking a fibre supplement. Drinking lots of quality water is good health sense anyway. I will address this later.

And yes, I know you've been waiting for it, here it is up front. I'm not shy and neither should you be. It's Chapter One and we're going to talk about Poop.

Poop

How often should we poop, and what colour and shape should it be?

Ideally, gut specialists believe that the normal range is pooping one to three times every day. Yes, every day. It's also ideal if you have a feeling of 'completion' or emptiness, after each poop. Poop is our body's way of really telling us what's going on in our system - and it's definitely worthwhile paying attention to this - because it could be an indication that something is very wrong - or very right - with your body and general health.

On the next page is a diagram called the Bristol Stool Scale. It is designed to show what healthy (and unhealthy) poop looks like.

If you just sit and then flush without checking out what you leave behind, it may benefit you to take a moment and check out what's in that toilet bowl, because it can give you some vital information about your health.

Ideally, your poop should be 3 or 4 on the scale.

What does it mean if you are 1,2,5,6 or 7? Or if it's pasty or difficult to clean off the toilet bowl? Of if you strain to pass? These fall into the unhealthy range.

Bristol Stool Scale

Type 1	Seperate hard lumps, like nuts (hard to pass)
Type 2	Sausage-shaped but lumpy
Type 3	Like a sausage but with cracks on it's surface
Type 4	Like a sausage or snake, smooth and soft
Type 5	Soft blobs with clear-cut edges (passed easily)
Type 6	Fluffy pieces with ragged edges, a mushy stool
Type 7	Watery, no solid pieces. Entirely liquid

Further unhealthy tips on what unhealthy poop may look like:
• Any poop that is narrow or ribbon-like can indicate some sort of bowel obstruction.

- Black, tarry or bright red - may indicate bleeding (black can also be an over-indulgence of licorice, some medications or supplements).
- White, pale or gray - may indicate a lack of bile, or something more serious (although if you take antacids this might impact the colour and make it pale. I don't take antacids as my research shows they just mask a problem, they don't fix it.)
- Floaters or poop that splashes can be an indication of some sort of inflammation.
- Undigested food is also not good (except for corn - more on this soon).
- It just really, really stinks (a mild smell is normal. A 'better not go in the bathroom for 15 minutes' type of stink indicates it's been inside you too long. And that isn't good. The longer it stays inside you, the more fluid your body extracts from it, and the harder it is to pass. And regular straining can lead to all sorts of unpleasantness.)

If your poop fits into any of these (or any other non-normal description on the Bristol Stool Scale), then it's worthwhile getting it tested. So see your doctor - particularly if it's been an issue for a while. There are all sorts of things that could be causing unhealthy poop - including ulcerative colitis, hepatitis, parasites (particularly if you've been travelling), inflammatory bowel disease, Crohn's disease, a malabsorption issue (that is, not getting your nutrients from your food), Cystic fibrosis and irritable bowel syndrome among others.

Another note I might add is how you sit on the loo, and how that can contribute to your digestive issues. By sitting on the loo the way we do, we scrunch up our descending colon (that's the bit that links to your rectum). This makes it MUCH more difficult for the waste product to move out of you and into the toilet bowl. The squat toilets, which you may have used while travelling, are really much healthier. There are two ways you can fix this - one is to move your body forwards and backwards while you're sitting on the loo. The other is to buy a footstool to raise your knees, thereby straightening out your colon.

Before you ask, yes, I have a footstool in my loo. So my feet are raised and my colon is straight. It really helps with a feeling of 'completeness' after my visit.

Oh, and what about flatulence? Yes, the good old fart. Well, a mild smelling fart is **completely normal**. Yep, completely. In fact, it's not only normal - it's desirable! Passing gas shows our gut bacteria are doing their job. We pass wind about 14 times a day - if we didn't, we'd blow up like balloons. That doesn't mean of course, that you just let fly any time you feel like it - social convention frowns on that - but do know that it's completely normal.

Constipation

What if you're regularly constipated? There are a number of lifestyle changes you can make that can help, including:

- You may be overdoing the fibre, so reduce fruits and vegetables
- Stress shows in our gut, so you might need to employ some stress management tactics (like meditation)
- Ignoring your body's cry for a loo visit can be a big contributor
- Not exercising enough - you need exercise to keep the gut moving
- Not enough water - yes, so much about our health comes down adequate hydration
- Calcium or iron supplements - do check that these are good for you
- Medication or over the counter drugs such as painkillers with codeine, antacids, or overuse of laxatives
- Food allergies can also contribute so it's worthwhile getting tested

Diarrhoea

What about constant diarrhoea? Well, there are some lifestyle changes you can make for that type of condition too.

- Increase your fruit and vegetable intake so you get more fibre (more vegetables than fruit, you don't want to overdo the fructose, or sugar, that is in fruit)
- Do more exercise
- Surprisingly, drink more water! Yes, there's that hydration issue again.
- Employ some stress management tactics (like meditation)
- Get checked out for food allergies

Beautiful food choices - they can make all the difference

I have pretty much eliminated most processed foods from my diet. I'm lucky that I have a wide range of fresh fruit and vegetable options where I live, and enjoy going to our local farm fresh shop, butcher and seafood stores. What it really means is that I make my meals from scratch and rarely eat takeaway food or pre-prepared frozen meals.

About 75 percent of the sugar we eat is 'hidden' in pre-made foodstuffs. So by cooking all my food myself, I automatically reduced my sugar intake, lowering the chances of gut inflammation and dehydrated skin cells. (To get a good idea of how much of a problem this is, check out *That Sugar Film* written and hosted by Australian Damon Gameau.)

You could do this too. If you are a city dweller and the supermarket is your closest option - then by all means, don't stop buying your fresh food there. And if you don't have time to make everything from scratch, there are some good options in prepared food. I'm talking about ready to cook fresh vegetables, rather than frozen meals (which I have never found tasty and they always smell funny. But if you enjoy them, then that may well be a better choice when you're in a hurry than a takeaway meal).

Did your mum always say to chew your food? Here's why...

When I started focusing on how I ate, I realised that I didn't chew my food enough before I swallowed. Not chewing enough placed an enormous strain on my stomach, as the stomach acid had to work super hard to get the food ready for its trip down my intestines. Even then, it can't do its job well enough sometimes. Some food will eventually filter through the intestinal wall, making its way into my blood stream. This is often called leaky gut and can cause all manner of problems.

The average meal takes between 18 and 72 hours to travel through your digestive system (depending on what you have eaten). So it pays to chew your food well so you don't get a digestive traffic jam.

I now chew each mouthful until it is seriously mashed up, almost liquified, and do you know what has happened? Several things really.

It takes me longer to eat a meal. Which means the message that I've eaten enough gets from my tummy to my brain. Which means I don't over eat; portion control is a big contributor to healthy eating and healthy weight.

I get more flavour from my food because I'm paying attention to it, so I am enjoying the sensation of eating more.

Sometimes, if I'm eating food with my hands and not cutlery, I eat with my left hand (I am right handed) as this helps to slow down eating.

I know being 'mindful' is the catch phrase of the moment - but it really is important to approach food this way. Really being aware of what you eat, rather than shoving it in your mouth at record speed will make a huge difference to your enjoyment of food, and your digestion - read health.

Love Your Liver

The human liver is the most extraordinary organ. It is the only internal organ that can regenerate itself - but there is a limit (think cirrhosis).

I'm not going to lecture about alcohol because I do love a glass of red wine. But the liver is so much more than a filtering system for booze. Your liver, in fact, performs over 500 functions. But don't worry, I won't list them all here.

Your liver decides how to manage the carbs, proteins and fats you eat. It decides how to process the components of food that are the building blocks of your bones, muscles, tissues, red blood cells - well, you get the idea.

Your liver might use some of the carbs, proteins and fats for energy or it might send some of them unchanged, straight into the bloodstream. It might tweak them a bit before sending them out into your blood, or it might store some of them for a while for later use.

Isn't that amazing! But no matter where in your body proteins, carbs and fats end up - they are processed by your liver.

So it makes sense to love your liver, doesn't it?! I take a pharmaceutical-grade liver supplement, that follows good manufacturing processes (not just something off the chemist or supermarket shelf) to make sure my liver is as healthy as it can be, and so far, so good, my liver function is top notch.

It may be because I had Hepatitis A when I was a young teenager and I have always been aware of liver health. It taught me how awful life can be if your liver isn't functioning properly - and I never want to experience something like that again.

Check in with me at meredith@meredithyardley.com to find out more about how you can go about supporting your liver.

Water, Water Everywhere

As I've outlined in this chapter, drinking at least eight glasses of water a day is really essential for your health. I've always loved water, so drinking eight glasses a day for me is no effort. But I have heard the complaints: 'it's boring', 'it's flavourless', 'it makes me want to pee too much'.

Suck it up, sunshine! Water cleanses you on the inside. It helps flush the liver and kidneys - and if these organs are congested it will show on your skin and on your face.

You could jazz it up a bit by making an infusion, using herbs, like mint, and fruit such as orange, berries or watermelon, or veggies such as cucumber or celery.

Be mindful of the water you drink too, for instance, tap can be water full of nasties, including heavy metals. And worse, much first world tap water contains fluoride, which was classified in 2014 by that highly regarded journal, *The Lancet*, as a neurotoxin. This puts fluoride in the same category as mercury and lead.

I use a bench top jug with a filter and use it for the kettle, veggies preparation and cooking, and making ice cubes. Other options are a reverse-osmosis or an alkaline filters. Do your research and figure out which suits you.

Another healthy skin trick is drinking a glass of warm lemon water in the morning. (Some dentists will say that the lemon water or apple cider vinegar can affect your tooth enamel. If that's a concern, you could use a straw, or rinse your mouth out or clean your teeth afterwards.) It's a wonderful cleanser and helps balance out the acid in your system.

I throw together a lemon (including pith and skin), a chunk of ginger and a teaspoon of organic turmeric into a blender, mix it all up, pop it in an ice cube tray and them make a pot of tea in the mornings.

What I don't drink warm I add in small amounts to my water during the day.

How big is a glass? About 250 ml, or a cup.

Best of all, water plumps up your cells, and plump cells don't wrinkle as much. So drinking water can have a surprising natural face-lifting effect. So, chin chin!

The Corn Test

It's a good idea to know how long your system takes to digest because you will discover how efficient your system is.

If you're not sure how long it takes your body to digest a meal, do the corn test.

Eat some corn, on the cob is best, and then keep an eye out for when it appears in your toilet bowl.

If it's longer than 24 hours before the first sighting then you have a sluggish system and this could be causing you problems.

Corn is a good choice because although the matter on the inside of the kernel breaks down, the outside doesn't, so it's easy to see.

(You can use beetroot if you don't like, or can't eat, corn.)

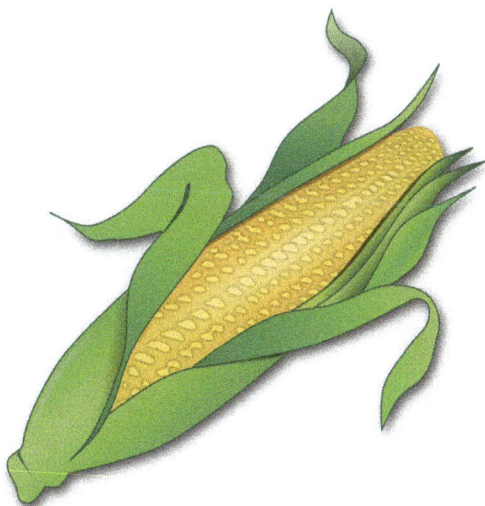

Chapter 2
Why do we wrinkle as we age?

'Inner beauty is priceless. Outer beauty doesn't
have to be.' - Paula Begoun

Your skin is your biggest organ. Really! But it's a lot more than that.

Your skin is the window to what's going on inside you. You radiate energy and glow when you are in love, when you are eating well, sleeping well, when you are full of energy and vitality, when your life is in balance.

But when you are suffering from sleep deprivation, stress, or the effects of smoking, drinking to excess, taking recreational drugs or making poor food choices (see Chapter 4), your skin shows it to the world by looking dull, tired and lacking in lustre.

Your skin is an extraordinary organ. It keeps bacteria and nasties out of your body and protects the organs, tissues, muscles on the inside. It is your very own radiator, helping to maintain your body temperature, and enabling you to experience sensation.

Here are some facts about your skin:
• Skin cells (on your skin's surface) renew themselves every 27-28 days.
• Your body is made up of 70 percent water, and 30 percent of it is in your skin.
• Your lips have fewer layers of skin than the rest of your face, so need a bit of extra sun protection.
• You shed around 18 kilos of skin in an average lifetime.
• The skin under your eyes is fragile, so it needs to be treated gently.
• Your skin has, at least, five sensation receptors that respond to pain and touch.

- Your skin accounts for 15 percent of your total body weight.
- The thinnest skin on your body is on your eyelids (0.02mm thick), the thickest is on the soles of your feet.
- The function of the skin is specific to its location - so the skin on your feet clearly has a different role than the skin on the back of your neck.
- It's an emotional barometer of your life.

Why do some of us look older than others?

I struggled with how much information to put into this chapter. Do you want to know the detail about each layer of your skin, how the cells move from the bottom to the top and what they do on the way?

I figured you might not have enough time to read such a detailed description. Just like me, you just want to know how to nourish and protect your skin. So I'll keep it simple and just share the basics.

You have three layers of skin. The bottom layer is the hypodermis, the middle layer is the dermis, and the epidermis is the layer everyone gets to see.

The hypodermis (the bottom layer looking at your skin from the outside in) contains sweat glands, fat, blood vessels, nerves, some hair follicles and oil glands.

The dermis (the middle layer) has blood vessels, nerves, hair follicles and oil glands, collagen and elastin. This layer provides the nutrients to the epidermis.

The top layer, the epidermis, contains the pigment and proteins.

Skin cells perform different functions as they move through the three layers. By the time the cells reach the top layer, the epidermis, they are nearly empty. They will spend about 27 days there, and eventually get sloughed off. (This is why exfoliating is so important - as we age our bodies become less efficient at sloughing off the dead skin, so exfoliating helps clean away space for the new cells coming to the top, keeping your skin 'breathing').

The important thing to know here is that it's not the top layer of cells, the epidermis, we are aiming at when we moisturise. These cells are already on their way out. It's the dermis layer we want to target which is where the collagen and elastin lie. Collagen and elastin are what keeps our skin tight and plump - helping us to keep a youthful look.

This is why choosing quality skin care (and not just for the face - but body moisturiser, bath and shower gel and hair products) is important.

Eating your way to beautiful skin

Eating quality foods that are full of vitamins, minerals and nutrients, drinking lots of water and avoiding dehydrating drinks such as excess coffee and alcohol are important to achieving and maintaining beautiful and youthful skin. You want to nourish those cells so they stay nice and plump and postpone you looking aged.

When you were born, your skin was über smooth. About age 25, your natural regenerative processes began to slow down. You probably wouldn't have noticed it - but it was there, and it continues as you age. Some of these processes are under your control, and some are not.

Factors such as genetics, exposure to the sun and other environmental damage, temperature extremes, pollution, stress, poor nutrition, excess skin dehydrators such as coffee, alcohol and smoking all contribute to the skin ageing.

And remember, it's not just your face that requires nutrients.

A good quality body cream will nourish those skin cells, plump them up and reduce fine lines.

We have all got the message about wearing a hat to protect our skin from the sun. Despite it giving us hat hair, it's still one of the best ways to protect our face from those damaging sun's rays. It helps with the important stuff of getting the sunshine you need - think Vitamin D - without the skin damage.

But what is the other part of your body where you get massive amounts of sun, and very few of us do anything to protect it?

Give up? It's your hands. Think about it. You use your hands every day in a myriad of ways, writing, washing up, carrying books, papers, children, shopping. And what is in the firing line for loads of sun when you drive? That's right - your hands.

So do yourself a favour and get some driving gloves. They are available at big department stores, or you can buy them online, they range from about US$10 to silly prices for those with aspirational labels. It doesn't matter what they are or how much you spend. Just get some to protect yourself from sunspots and freckles.

But of course, our face, neck, décolletage and our arms show our age too. What do you look for in a moisturiser? Or don't you think about it much?

I look for very specific things. Firstly, flick anything that has a long list of chemicals (you can find out more in my Bonus Chapter - *Is Your Skin Care a Health Hazard?* All the details on how to get a copy are at the front of the book).

Secondly, look for products that are botanically based. Products with loads of vitamins, such as Vitamins A, B, C, E are good. These vitamins are vital to our health, and as you have already realised, these will pass through your skin into your cells, organs, tissues, and muscles.

I also look for a skin care with self-preserving technology because I don't want any of those nasty preservatives in my skin care and on my skin.

You can make life easy for yourself, of course, and check out www.enrichyourenergy.usana.com to see what I use, or you can get in touch with me and we can have a chat about it – meredith@meredithyardley.com. The QR codes are below.

You can also watch this video and see what highly-regarded consulting dermatologist and physician Dr Regina Hamlin recommends.

Then you can see what I use, and order your own divine skin care!

Email me to chat about my skin care routine:

Chapter 3
Why wearing makeup to bed can make you look old

'Tomorrow is a new day; begin it well and serenely and with too high a spirit to be encumbered with your old nonsense.' - Ralph Waldo Emerson

Once upon a time I didn't fuss too much with my skin. Then age started to catch up with me and I thought I should do something, reasonably regularly.

I was travelling a lot for work, so I bought a packet of those face wipes. They seemed okay, were light in my luggage, and I felt I was at least doing *something*.

Then one day a colleague and I were preparing for a large presentation in front of about 300 people. And he committed a cardinal sin. He wrote on the white board with a permanent marker!

If you've ever been preparing for something big, and something really went screwy, you'll know how I was feeling. I needed to fix this fast!

Then I had a brilliant idea. I took out one of my face wipes and, voila! It removed the permanent marker.

And then it hit me. If this wipe could remove permanent marker from the whiteboard, what on earth was it doing to my skin?

The benefits of a regular beauty routine

Do you have a morning beauty routine? Or do you just slap some moisturiser on, swipe on a bit of lippy and blush and race off to your day?

At the end of your day, do you cleanse your face? Tone? Moisturise? Treat the skin under your eyes to something a bit nourishing? After all, that is where those bags will develop if you're not careful.

And what about exfoliating your face and body, or using a facial mask regularly?

I hear your pain. Time. Kids. Work. House. Partner. Sport. It all just seems so much easier to collapse into bed when you finally have the chance.

'Why go to all this trouble?' I hear you ask.

Every day we are exposed to pollution, smoke, radiation from electronics, sun damage and other environmental factors. Our skin deals with all this as well as our lack of sleep, occasional poor diet choices, stress and even free radicals.

Even more detrimental to the skin are the three big ones - smoking and the overuse of alcohol and coffee. Too much coffee and alcohol can suck the moisture right out of your skin - and you know what that means. Collagen damage and wrinkles.

I enjoy a coffee a day - just one. And I like a glass of red wine with my dinner. But in my view, and in the view of thousands of medical and health professionals, there is no safe level of smoking. So if you smoke and you want good skin - just know you can't have both. You're going to have to choose. Please choose wisely.

But back to the beauty routine. It doesn't need to take a long time - you really can do it in a few minutes a day. Twice a week you can include an exfoliation; and then three times a month (or more if you want) enjoy a facial mask.

Caring for your face isn't a burden. It's a little way that you, every day, can show you care about yourself. If you have kids, it makes for a great role model behaviour.

Do you want your daughter or son to put themselves last all the time because they are emulating their mother? Really, you owe it to your kids to show them looking after themselves is an important part of being human.

I still put myself last in the greater scheme of loved ones, sometimes. But I'm a lot better than I was, and now I MAKE time for me. And the more I do it, the more enjoyable it becomes.

I feel nourished and nurtured because I look after me.

After all, the safety procedures on airlines always say fit your face mask first before looking after others - and there's a reason for this. We just CAN'T look after other people properly unless we are looking after ourselves.

Just think about it for a minute (because I know you probably only just have a minute or two right now to spend time thinking about YOU).

Close your eyes and imagine these three things: (yes I know you can't close your eyes and read at the same time, just work with me here! :))

1. You wake refreshed after having a good night's sleep.
2. Your face is glowing because you have been using quality skin care in your beauty routine for a few weeks.

3. You've upped your nutrition and your insides are behaving - no bloating, no indigestion, no reflux, and you are having regular, and successful, visits to the smallest room in the house.

Then imagine a friend or family member needs your help with something, like taking on extra 'mum's taxi' trips to your kid's sporting event; writing a project report for a colleague who's swamped; working an extra day. It could even be stepping in to help your favourite charity because another member is sick or stepping up, stepping forward, helping out anywhere.

How much more **energy** do you think you'd have to help them if you have just these three things under control? I'll wager you'd have loads - and you'd not just have the energy to help. You'd also have no resentment or feelings of overwhelm about being asked, because you know you can cope.

Only through being yourself can you give to the others in your world your greatest gifts. To do any less betrays both them and yourself - Ken Carey

So in reality, by looking after yourself, you're doing a community service!

Just a quick note: Learning to say 'NO' is also a really good thing to incorporate into your life. Check out Chapter 6 for some ways you can learn to say no without feeling guilty.

Now, let's look at the beauty routine itself. It takes far less time than you think. Let me show you:

Morning:
Do you shower in the morning? Then have your cleanser in the shower, apply when you first get in (remembering your neck and decolletáge), and by the time you wash your hair, your cleanser will

have done its work and be ready to be washed off, just with your hands.

After you dry off, apply your toner, wait for it to dry, (do something else to get ready like brush or blow dry your hair), then apply your SPF 15+ moisturiser (again, remembering your neck and decolletáge). When you've finished drying off, apply your body moisturiser to legs and arms. Total time? Three minutes - max.

If you don't shower in the morning, just follow the cleanse, tone, moisturise routine. Oh, and if your moisturiser doesn't contain sunscreen, then find a good quality sunscreen and use it on your face, decolletáge, and the back of your hands.

Evening:
If you shower at night, then just follow the above.

Cleanse, and wash off the cleanser with a clean face cloth, or use those cute little sponges (just make sure they dry properly before storing them as they can mould if stored wet). Tone - as above and then moisturise with a night cream.

Remember also to moisturise your arms and legs (particularly when you have the 'crocodile skin' look going - your skin is dry, so nourish it, it needs a bit of loving).

Does this mean you should cleanse, tone and moisturise twice a day?

YES!

Cleansing etc.. at the end of the day is a no-brainer. But what many people don't understand is what happens to our skin as we sleep.

Resting is good for our bodies and our minds, but our skin works overtime during sleeping, renewing, recovering and replenishing during the nighttime hours.

I have created a short video so you can see how I cleanse, tone and moisturise my skin twice a day (don't worry, you won't have to watch me in the shower!)

MY SKIN CARE ROUTINE

If you want to do what I do, there are a couple more steps.

Every day I use an eye nourisher below my eyes. Why? This skin is very delicate under your eyes and has much less oil to keep it fresh so it needs a bit extra tender loving care.

Gently apply a teeny bit to the tip of one of your ring fingers, tap your other ring finger to share the cream, then gently - **very gently** - pat the cream along your ocular bone below your eye (that's the edge of the eye socket), starting from the outside and moving to the inside. Going from out to in means you don't stretch the skin.

I always use an essence on my face in the morning, to plump up those cells to look smoother. And every second evening I use a serum to really penetrate the skin. Essences and serums provide special treatments to nourish and beautify your skin, and provide antioxidant protection. They are an extra, so if your budget only stretches to good quality basic skin care, choose that. A good base is much better, and more protective, for your skin than an entire range of poorer quality product.

I also use an exfoliant twice a week. Exfoliation is a key step in skin care because it helps to remove accumulated dead skin and dirt that can irritate your skin, build up into little spots, and take away your glow.

I cleanse my face in the shower, then wash myself and my hair, and then, just before I have finished showering, I exfoliate my face. Why at the end of the shower? Because even with just a warm shower the pores of my face have opened just that little bit extra and the gentle exfoliator can remove some of the deeper grime and gunk.

Your face doesn't need to be scrubbed. It's not going to the gym. Just a gentle, circular almost patting motion is sufficient. If your skin is red, it's likely you've been too enthusiastic about it. Try to be more gentle next time.

Two or three times a month I treat myself to a beautiful deep, enriching, white clay facial mask. I cleanse, exfoliate, then apply the masque. It takes about 20 minutes to do its magic, and then I wash it off. Then I apply essence or serum, eye nourisher and moisturise.

I have followed this routine for three years now and I can't remember the last time I had a blackhead, whitehead or breakout.

Not only that, recently I was at the beautician (getting an eyebrow and eyelash tint - the curse of being very fair is that I have no eye definition!) and the young beautician remarked she'd love to upsell me on their products, but couldn't because my skin was in such good shape. She then asked me all sorts of questions about what I used and when I used it. I left that treatment feeling pretty good!

If you have rosacea, dermatitis, eczema, dermatitis, psoriasis, seborrhea or other skin conditions, you might be better to seek advice from a dermatologist.

The nitty gritty about serums and essences, what they are and how they differ.

What is a serum? A serum is generally rich in alpha-hydroxy or beta-hydroxy acid-based components. Some use both alpha and beta.

Alpha-hydroxy is a glycol acid that penetrates the skin, loosens the bonds between the dead skin cells so they are more easily removed. As well, their molecules bind to water, keeping your cells plumper. This gives your skin a smooth, vibrant appearance. Alpha-hydroxy can be found in things like sugar cane, lactic acid (found in milk), malic acid (found in apples) and tartaric acid (found in grapes). By loosening the link between the dead keratin, alpha-hydroxy acids act as exfoliants.

Beta-hydroxy is salicylic acid, which is also an exfoliant. Salicylic acid has a deep cleansing capability, which can prepare your skin for the nourishment of the quality moisturiser you apply in the next step of your skin care routine.

Serums are not appropriate for every skin type and should be used gently and sparingly at first to ensure you have no reaction. You could try them on the inside of your wrist at first to see if there is any reaction.

What is an essence? An essence is different to a serum, as it contains no alpha or beta hydroxy acids. Rather it generally contains amino acids and humectants that help build the skin tissue. Some essences are really well made and can help reduce fine lines, sun spots, and the appearance of damaged skin.

Both serums and essences are designed to refine and renew your skin. But give it time – it's taken you a number of years to get these blemishes, it will take some time for the quality skin care to do its job removing them. Skin care is a lifetime commitment, so bring a long term focus and you'll see pleasing changes over time.

Besides looking and feeling good, there is another, more esoteric reason to have a beauty routine.

A beauty routine is more than just a beauty routine - it is a ritual in which a woman - YOU - can add very personal meaning to your day. I talk more about the importance of routine and rituals in Chapter 6, but until then….

Honour yourself by looking after yourself

Make Up

Just a quick note about makeup.

I don't use much. As you can see from my photos, I am fair, so I usually get just a lash and eyebrow tint and eyebrow wax.

When I need more definition for my eyes, I use a mascara. I have an organic blush, and I use an organic lip stick. I buy all my makeup from a health food store. I just don't trust the big brands.

Skin Care Product Checklist

What skin care do I use? Well, you can click here to find out more about my preference.

My guiding principles are:

- Always buy the best quality you can afford.

- Choose products that have a botanical base.

- Use a day moisturiser that has at least an SPF factor 15. If you want more coverage try a mineral foundation.

- Choose products that are dripping with good quality vitamins and other minerals to nourish your skin's cells. Good starting points are:
  - Vitamin C assists collagen production and improves skin tone and smoothness.
  - Vitamin A helps with healing and creating new skin tissue.
  - Vitamin E is an antioxidant that helps protect against free radical damage.
  - Zinc helps repair and strengthen tissue.
  - Grapeseed extract is a highly potent antioxidant to protect the skin.
  - Beta carotene helps maintain the integrity of all cell membranes and your digestive system.
  - Omega 3s help feed the cells, keeping them plump.

- Choose products that have independent scientific evidence behind them, proving they do what they say they do. Ask to see the results and if they can't show the results, then really, think twice about using the product.

- Choose products that have no chemical nasties. That includes looking for BHP-free packaging.

- Choose products that have packaging that protects the product - i.e. that you don't stick your finger or applicator in - this will ensure no bacteria enters the product.

- Check that the packaging is treated so it can't leak into your product, and visa versa.

- Choose a product provider that makes the product themselves, not someone that engages a third party to make it and then just slaps their label on it. That way you can be sure that what is on the ingredients list is actually what the manufacturer has put in the product.

Chapter 4
Food and nutrition for beautiful skin

'Symptoms are a way for your body to say, 'Listen to me talk for a change'.' - Carl A Hammerschlag

I'm sure you've heard the saying 'You are what you eat'. I like what Sue Ward (nutritionist at the Sanoviv Medical Institute) says: 'You are what you eat, digest and absorb'.

And it's never more true than eating for glowing skin.

'The skin is the last organ to receive nourishment from the body, and the first to show signs of nutritional deficiency, imbalance or illness,' says Dr. Regina Hamlin, consulting dermatologist in the United States.

Superfoods for your Skin

Feeding your skin from the inside is really quite easy. Here is a quick checklist of foods that you would benefit from including regularly in your diet.

* Fresh (organic and free range if you can) meat, chicken, and eggs.

* Toss out the sweeteners for your coffee and tea - including sugar, malt extract and chemical sweeteners. If you need a bit of sweetening in your tea or coffee, try organic Manuka honey - it is good for you and has proven healing qualities. Or try Stevia powder - it's a natural plant extract and you need less of it than sugar.

- Fresh fruit is berry good for you! Puns aside, berries are a brilliant antioxidant food that help build cell health. I buy loads when they are in season, using some and throwing some into the freezer for when they aren't in season so I have them all year round.

- Use fresh herbs, and lots of them. Don't just use them for garnish, include them in the meal itself. Parsley, which cleans the blood and helps the breath, sage with chicken, mint is particularly good in your water with lemon and cucumber....

- Fats: include Omega 3s in your diet. You can get these from fish oils, flax seeds, nuts, avocados and olives.

    - Eat oily fish, such as salmon or tuna, three times a week. These are high in omega-3 fatty acids DHA and EPA which give you the double benefits of glowing skin, and protecting your cells from early ageing.

    - Use extra virgin olive oil, coconut oil, butter, avocados, olives, nuts and tahini.

    - Best of all - a single square of 85 percent dark chocolate is choc-full (sorry!) of antioxidants

What are DHA and EPA? DHA = Docosahexaenoic and EPA = Eicosapentaenoic. These are acids high in Omega-3 that are vital to maintaining a healthy function throughout our bodies including the brain, retina, cardiovascular system, human growth and intellectual development. So pretty important stuff.

What fats to avoid

Transfats are on the top of the list. They include margarine, canola and safflower oils. Why should we avoid them? Many doctors consider transfats the worst kind as they push up your bad cholesterol (LDL) and lower your good cholesterol (HDL).

Now some animal products (meat and dairy) contain small amounts of transfats, but these are naturally occurring and don't amount to too much (like anything, however, these can be over-represented in a diet).

The real danger of transfats is in processed foods. They're used to contribute to taste, and give foods a longer shelf life. They also mean some restaurants can used partially hydrogenated vegetable oil in their deep fryers so they don't need to change the oil as frequently as they would with other oils.

Foods where you'll find transfats (known as 'partially hydrogenated' oil) include:
• baked goods: cakes, cookies, pies, crackers, ready-made frosting
• snacks such as potato and corn chips, and some popcorn
• fried foods: french fries, donuts, fried chicken
• refrigerator dough such as canned biscuits and frozen pizza
• coffee creamer and margarine.

Really, if you have a little treat every now and then, that's okay (because I know you're human, just like me and sometimes we need a little treat just to help us manage through the day), but please, don't make these things a regular part of your diet.

Other ideas

When I worked in the corporate world, I would cook a soup in a slow cooker over the weekend (it would make my apartment smell fabulous!). Preparation doesn't take long, and the cooking time is left to the slow cooker, or crock pot, so I could go off and do other things.

Then I would freeze my soup in handy little containers and take them to work - still frozen. By the time lunch came around, they had mostly defrosted so I could microwave them and have a wholesome lunch.

Just as an aside, I know some people don't hold with microwaves. I am not one of them. I think they are brilliant devices that can make one's life super easy by giving back some time. And, being time poor as I know you are, microwaves can make a huge difference to a healthy diet.

In summer, making up a basic salad and leaving it in the fridge undressed gives you two or three days worth of lunch and/or dinner.

To avoid boring yourself with the same food, you can change each meal by adding nuts (walnuts, almonds); or orange, lemon or lime zest and juice; or another vegetable, or fruit, such as an apple, pear or peach; or a mixture of the above as well as mint, coriander, basil, lemon or parsley. Then by adding different meats, legumes or an egg, you can change a simple salad into something new and fresh each meal.

I have some favourite vegetables that I use in several different ways. Zucchini is my all time favourite veg - you can grate it into a salad or omelette, stir fry it, barbecue it, make noodles out of it, open grill it with garlic and a small amount of olive oil, steam it or roast it.

I also love sweet potato (kumera), because I believe we eat with our eyes and the orange is such an attractive addition to a plate. It's also delicious, and it, too, can be cooked so many different ways, including stir fry, mashing, baking with orange and a bit of brown sugar (just a bit!), wrapping in foil and barbecuing. It works well with fresh orange juice and zest, and is sensational mashed with fresh ginger.

Another favourite is tomato - and the list of what you can do with tomatoes is endless. Peel, poach, bake, slow cook, chop in a salad or salsa, use as a base for a winter stew - you are only limited by your imagination.

Asparagus. Yum. Super yum lightly steamed, and served with a little bit of cold pressed olive oil and parmesan or pecorino cheese sprinkled over the spears. You can also char grill asparagus, or just chop in a bowl, pour boiling water over the spears and let them steep for a few minutes (depending on how much 'crunch' you like) and then rinse them in cold water to stop them cooking. Use in a stir fry, omelette, salad, or just as a simple side dish.

But you might not have time to do that all the time. And I get that. So if you go to a supermarket - skip the pre-packaged frozen foods and get some fresh meat (or a cooked chicken), some prepared vegetables or salad and use those to create a meal. It's not perfect, but it's practical, it's pragmatic, and it's a good alternative for a healthy meal.

Refined Sugars

Have a look at your pantry and your fridge and think about what you really have there. I'm not trying to stop you enjoying the occasional treat, but if you regularly eat crackers, chips and other snack foods, you are not doing yourself any favours.

Go to your fridge and freezer and get rid of anything that is in packaging, including fast or frozen meals (keep the ones you've cooked and frozen yourself of course)

I guess you've heard a bit about ditching the sugar, about it being the enemy and no good for you. Well, some sugars ARE good for you. But you won't find them in processed foods. You'll only find the good sugars in fruits and vegetables you cook for yourself.

How do you know if an item has a load of hidden sugar? It often has 'low fat', 'fat free' or 'reduced fat' on its label. 'Fat is flavour', any chef will tell you that, and if you take away the fat, you are left with yuck - so to make the yuck taste good, food manufacturers replace the fat with sugar or sugar substitute like high fructose corn syrup.

But why is refined sugar so bad for us? Here are a few reasons why excessive sugar is the enemy of good health and why it's such a contributor to fast ageing:

1. It spikes your hormones. Sugar contributes massively to mood and energy highs and lows. It can also disrupt one of the most powerful hormones in your body - insulin. Insulin is your fat storing hormone, and is a link to all other hormones in your body, including oestrogen and testosterone, so imbalances in these hormones can be caused by eating sugar.

2. Inflammation. Excessive sugar can be responsible for much of the inflammation in our bodies, and this can truly be deadly. Refined sugar-heavy diets put strain on the heart because they increase the level of oxidative stress in your system.

3. It's sneaky. Sugar hides everywhere. It's in pasta sauce, yoghurt, iced tea, breakfast bars. It's going to be in anything that has low, reduced, or no fat on the label, because you have to replace the flavour of fat with something, and food manufacturers have decided that something is going to be sugar. Or worse, it's replaced with high fructose corn syrup (HFC) (and if it's from the US it's probably genetically modified corn - but that's another story). HFC is now being relabelled in the United States as plain old fructose or 'natural sweetener', and is derived from GMO corn. It's designed to make the consumer oblivious to what they are eating. So be careful, and learn to read labels. Or just don't buy processed food.

4. Research is now discovering fat isn't the cause of fat - excess and refined sugar is the culprit. Following on from point number 1, when your body gets refined sugars it doesn't use them the way it does complex sugars (such as the sugars in vegetables). So it stores them, and this leads to insulin spikes and the storing of fat.

5. Understanding the Glycemic Index is the best way to learn about sugars. We have the world leading Low Glycemic Index Institute right here in Australia at the University of Sydney. So check out www.glycemicindex.org, and find out how to identify those foods that are high in sugar and those that are low in sugar so you can make better, more informed choices, and you'll be on your way to a healthier you.

Nutritional Supplements - are they really necessary?

By now you know it's not just through skin products that I look after my skin. As you've seen, diet plays a huge part.

But I believe nutritional supplements are also a necessity. Why? Because, with modern farming practices, we just don't get the vitamins and minerals from our food the way our grandparents did when they were young.

If you have no interest in what's in your food, or the conditions of its production, and where it comes from, by all means skip this section.

But before you do, just think about a couple of things: Where do you get your minerals from? Without minerals, you can't absorb the vitamins that are in your food.

I'm not the only one. The Journal of the American Medical Association (JAMA) recently reversed a long-standing anti-vitamin stance by publishing two scientific review articles recommending that multivitamin supplements should be taken by all adults as a general rule.

Modern Farming

In 1950, you could get 4.3mg of iron from one apple, today you need to eat 26 apples to get 0.18mg of iron. And you need to eat eight oranges now to get the same amount of Vitamin A that your grandparents (in the early 20th century) got from one orange.

At the 1992 Rio Earth Summit, findings were released that confirmed topsoil depletion existed across the globe through the 20th century. Over this time, US and Canada's agricultural soils lost 85 percent of their mineral content, Asian and South American soils lost 76 percent, while Africa, Europe and Australia lost 74 percent. Without robust topsoil, we don't get the minerals we need in our foods.

According to the *Institute for Optimum Nutrition*, the minerals in our fruits and vegetables have depleted over time. This is their table of mineral loss recorded between 1940-1991:

Mineral	Vegetables	Fruit
Sodium	-49%	-29%
Potassium	-16%	-19%
Magnesium	-24%	-16%
Calcium	-46%	-16%
Iron	-27%	-24%
Copper	-76%	-20%
Zinc	-59%	-27%

source: ion.ac.uk

And although these figures are from a 2006 article, let's face it, our farming practices have hardly improved.

Once upon a time farmers would move to new farming lands, or replenish the soil with organic waste when the soils were spent. They also turned the soil which had organic matter in it. Today, the same land is used over and over again, for the same crops. A significant amount of pesticides and herbicides are also used, which depletes soil even further.

So unless you grow your own vegetables and fruit, in an organic setting, with no possible infection from other local farmers who aren't organic - the chances of you getting the amount of minerals and vitamins you need for a healthy body are pretty slim.

What does Recommended Daily Allowance REALLY mean?

Do you know? People do go on about Recommended Daily Allowance (RDA) or Recommended Daily Intake (RDI) as if there is some major scientific meaning for it. In one way there is. But probably not in the way you think.

RDA's were developed in the 1930s (and were changed a little bit later), to reduce the incidence of scurvy, rickets and pellagra (pellagra is a vitamin deficiency with some nasty consequences). They represent a *minimum* number, to protect against some pretty specific problems.

But if you are relying on today's RDA's to guard against degenerative disease, such as diabetes, heart disease or stress, you'll be sorely disappointed. The Medical Research Education Associates website says it better than I can:

'Today, we live in a sea of pollution. Air pollution, contaminated sources of water, radiation, over-processed foods, soils that are depleted of their critical trace elements,

countless new toxic chemicals every month, and more and more prescriptive drugs. Couple these factors with less than adequate lifestyles and growing levels of psychological and physical stress, and you can see why the AMA report recommends supplements for virtually everyone.'

The Importance of Minerals in Your Diet

Okay, just a quick bit of information here to help you understand the importance of minerals in your diet. For ease, I'll just take the minerals mentioned in the table in the Modern Farming section:

- **Sodium**: (electrolyte) is essential to help regulate the right balance of fluids in your body. It assists in transmitting nerve impulses and helps with muscle control (such as contraction and relaxation). It also controls blood pressure and blood volume.

- **Potassium**: (electrolyte) maintains electrolyte balance in your body's cells, supports tissue function by helping send nerve impulses. It helps muscle control, helps release energy from protein, fat and carbohydrates, assists with waste removal and helps deliver oxygen to your brain.

- **Magnesium**: (electrolyte) essential for your heart health as it helps your heart muscles function better. It helps protect blood vessels and is a natural blood thinner and surprisingly enough, it assists with bowel movements.

- **Calcium**: (electrolyte) as well as assisting with bone health, calcium is important for muscle contraction, which includes your heart. It also assists with the release of hormones and enzymes, and help blood vessels move blood around your body.

- **Iron**: essential to help make red blood cells. Red blood cells carry oxygen around your body. (Not everyone needs a lot of iron - if you have any concerns about your iron content, ask your doctor for a blood test.)

- **Copper**: as well as working with iron to make red blood cells, copper helps keep blood vessels, nerves, and bones healthy, and supports your immune system.

- **Zinc**: is needed to help our immune system stay strong. Zinc also helps in cell health - cell division, cell growth, healing wounds. It also helps break down carbohydrates.

Is it Really Organic?

Eating truly organic produce is a great step towards getting all the vitamins and minerals we need. However there are different criteria applied by different countries when applying the term 'organic' that make it a bit difficult to have faith in the label that says 'organic'.

According to the United States Department of Agriculture (USDA), organic labelling must be certified, but up to five percent of non-organic ingredients (excluding salt and water) may be contained in the product (another reason to only buy fresh produce as much as possible.)

Further, in an example given on the USDA website, someone making a muffin mix combining organic and non-organic ingredients, can claim 'made with organic ingredients' status if 70 percent of the ingredients is certified organic. That means 30 percent of the product doesn't need to be organic to be labelled organic. And that 30 percent could contain some nasty pesticides and herbicides. And even genetically modified foodstuff can be included without your knowledge.

The European Union has tough criteria on organic produce, but still allows for chemical pesticides, fertilisers and antibiotics. Their website says they have 'strict limitations', as well as strict limits on food additives and processing aids.

So it would seem that organic is open to interpretation.

And this is why I choose to eat mainly whole foods (in that I buy the produce and cook it myself), and why I take a top-of-the-range pharmaceutical-grade, athlete-quality supplement. Because even with buying the best, organic food straight from the farmer, I know the soil is depleted to the point where I'm just not getting the vitamins and minerals I need from my food.

So there you have it. I enhance my diet with the highest quality supplements I can find, and I know my health has improved over the past few years because of it. If you are interested in using what I use, go to www.enrichyourenergy.usana.com, or connect with me at meredith@meredithyardley.com.

WHAT I USE

E-MAIL ME

Chapter 5
Loving yourself

'Twenty years from now you will be more disappointed by the things you didn't do than by the ones you did. So throw off the bowlines. Sail away from the safe harbour. Catch the trade winds in your sails. Explore. Dream. Discover.' - Mark Twain

And I would like to add a bit to Mark Twain's quote -

Explore, Dream, Discover YOURSELF!

In the end, this is what this book is really about. Looking after yourself, caring for yourself. Because **YOU** are really important. There are people in your life who love you, people who care about you, people who rely on you. Most directly, they are your parents, siblings, partners, children, colleagues and friends. Indirectly they are all the people that your parents, siblings, partners rely on too.

Look further afield, and they are the local service station where you buy your petrol, the corner store owner, your health professional, your sports team, your children's teachers, your colleagues. The list is endless.

There are many things you can do that see you looking after yourself. Some are small things in themselves, but together they create a much bigger whole.

And that whole is **YOU!**

What Can Water Tell Us?

Have you heard of Dr Masaru Emoto? He was a truly original thinker. Dr Emoto did some groundbreaking research on water.

How is that relevant you ask? Well, we humans are pretty much made up of water - so pay attention, this is super-relevant.

Dr Emoto did extensive research of water from around our plant. He realized that water shows its true form in its crystallized state, and that water is deeply connected to our collective consciousness. Sounds a bit weird? You just haven't seen the photos yet. Yes! He photographed water crystals that show beautiful patterns when the water undergoes things like being exposed to Bach's Goldberg Variations, or when a note that says 'Thank You' is taped to a bottle with water in it.

When the water is exposed to things like heavy metal music, or the words 'Adolf Hitler', the crystals are not crystalline at all - rather they are chaotic and fragmented.

You might argue that we bring that interpretation to the water in our perception of heavy metal music and our feelings about Adolf Hitler. And that could be true. But it's not the point. The water picks up the vibrations. And we are 70 percent water.

Dr Emoto's work showed water is alive and responsive. His research indicated we can use our own self nourishment to enjoy some self healing - and that this can expand to include others. Doesn't that sound lovely?

(To learn more - and there is so much more to explore, check out his books *Messages from Water, The Hidden Messages in Water* and *The True Power of Water.* You can also have a look at this short video.)

DR. EMOTO

Move - shake that booty any way you can!

Just MOVE! Every day, in every way you can. Get up from that desk every 45 minutes. Park at the far edge of the shopping centre carpark. Take the stairs wherever possible.

Walk in the local park or botanic gardens on a weekend or in the evening. Even better is if you can walk with a friend - time just flies. Incorporate walking into your everyday activities. Mix it up so it is enjoyable - that really is the key.

Walking is a wonderful exercise. It is free and you can walk at any time of the day or night (within limits of course). Conventional wisdom is to aim for 10,000 steps a day, but it's fine if you want to work up to that. Use a pedometer or one of the new-fangled wristbands (that's what I have - it makes walking fun because I get a little vibration when I hit 10,000 steps. It brings out my competitive nature and I walk just to feel it). The fact is that you will only achieve what you measure.

Walking also stimulates the lymphatic drainage system, which is our body's waste elimination system. And no-one wants a waste elimination system that's blocked up!

New science is pointing to sitting being the new smoking - the damage to our bodies from sitting for hours at a time is only just starting to be realised. It's not that sitting is necessarily bad for you, it's just that sitting tends to be a sedentary activity that can easily be overdone.

Dr James Levine, director of the Mayo Clinic-Arizona State University Obesity Solutions Initiative says, "Sitting is more dangerous than smoking, kills more people than HIV and is more treacherous than parachuting. *We are sitting ourselves to death.*"

Wow. Take a moment and think about that.

How much time do you spend sitting, in the car or on the train or bus? At work or at a computer at home. When you are watching TV and watching kids' sport. Add it up - you might be surprised.

Movement is also essential for beautiful skin. It gets the blood pumping, activates your lymphatic system, makes you want to drink water, and staves off early ageing.

A great way to start, or end, the day is with yoga. Really yoga is just stretching, so if it helps to think of it that way, go right ahead! I favour two yoga apps for my daily practice, DailyYoga, and YogaStudio. They're not expensive, and you can do your stretching wherever you are - hotel rooms, bedroom or loungeroom.

And even better, my friend Anne, who is a yoga and meditation teacher and food coach, shows you how to do office yoga! Check out her video here! (and she has a free ebook to give you too).

Moving regularly is essential, and incidental movement is just as beneficial as scheduled exercise.

Breathe

Breathe - it's free!

Mindful or conscious breathing has amazing health benefits. I'm not talking about the auto-pilot breathing we do every day.

I'm talking about 'mindful', or deliberate breathing. For instance, take three deep breaths before eating your meal. It will quieten your mind, and ready your body for the intake of food.

Whenever you start to feel yourself entering an emotional high or low - such as becoming angry, anxious, frustrated, sad, follow this five part recipe:

1. **Sit (or lie) somewhere quiet and close your eyes.**

2. **Take your hands and place them on your lower belly, below your navel.**

3. **Breathe in for a count of 5, deep down into your diaphragm. Your hands should move out with your belly.**

4. **Breathe out for a count of 6. Your hands should move in with your belly.**

5. **Repeat ideally for 20 breaths but if you can only do five, then that's a great start.**

Practice this breathing daily.

When you do 'mindful' breathing, your parasympathetic nervous system will be engaged. This is the part of your nervous system that calms you down and is the part of the human nervous system that kicked in with our cavemen ancestors when they were safe. All the scary creatures were somewhere else and they could relax around the river bank, or in the cave, knowing they didn't have to be on high alert.

The other part of our nervous system, the sympathetic nervous system, is our flight, fight or freeze mechanism. This is what we used, as cavemen, when we were hunting or under threat. This is where soldiers live when they are in battle. This is where many women live trying to be everything to everybody.

Constantly being in this state can make you very ill. It can even kill you, slowly though. It can lead to a stroke, or heart attack, or other stress-related or autoimmune-related conditions. This is NOT what you want.

What state do you live in?

Learn to breathe.

Reflect

Do you keep a diary? Or is it too much trouble? Keeping a diary has a lot of benefits, but I understand if your days are just too full to have the energy to write when you go to bed at night, or wake in the morning.

Diary keeping is a good way to keep yourself focused, and to have a little 'me' time. I know a lot of people who focus on the negatives when they write in their diaries. You know, the troubles they are having, the problems that won't go away. By writing down the negatives, you are emphasising them, focusing on them. And the more you focus on something, the more of it you will get!

What if you focused on writing just ONE thing you are grateful for before you go to bed. Or before you rise and meet your day.

Do it now.

Grab a piece of paper, and think about something you are truly thankful for. Not some response you *think* might be right but something real, deep down inside you.

The smell of your child's hair after they've bathed. Coming into the bedroom and seeing your husband has made the bed because he knows it's important to you. The daily smile from the barista at the coffee shop. These little things that we often stop noticing are the spiritual grease to our daily wheel.

My experience of diary keeping is quite profound. Without it, I wouldn't have found my husband, chucked in my corporate life and I definitely wouldn't be writing this book! Being clear about your life can help you manifest what you want. And it needs to be written down.

These small things are NOT small.

It's not the number of things you are grateful for that's important, and it's not the length of the sentence. It's the connection you have with what you are writing.

It's easy to write empty lists about being grateful for a roof over your head, an income, a reliable car. Of course, these are things to be grateful for, to appreciate, but it's more than that. Recognising what you are grateful for can be deeply fulfilling, and give you significant benefits across many areas of your life, including your psychological, social and physical health.

A specific gratitude diary can create amazing outcomes. First, you are focusing on the good stuff, not the bad stuff. Second, when you read it, your mind expands with all the great things you have in life.

Can you imagine how your life would lift if these were the last thoughts you had at night, or the first thoughts of your new day?

Yes, it takes work, particularly if things aren't going well. But it's like anything you do often, you get better at it. There is ALWAYS something to be grateful for, and once you start to recognise what these things are, the more you will see them.

Even if you hate your job, you had a lousy day, or you lost your house keys, you can be grateful you've just had that cup of coffee that tasted so good. It doesn't have to be a BIG gratitude; it just has to be acknowledged.

This is not to be confused with the Positive or Happiness Industry. I am not suggesting you go out and be Pollyanna when life is crap.

Treat yourself. Go to a stationery shop, or look online, and buy a journal that appeals to you. Make it pretty. Or decorative. Or geometrically crazy. Whatever sings to your soul. Use it to reflect on your life; use it to acknowledge appreciation; use it to create the life you want. You'll be amazed at the outcome.

What I am suggesting is that **gratitude, thankfulness, appreciation** is something that works at a deep level in our subconscious, and starts to expand our mind, and heart, helping us to find life more fulfilling. And fulfillment is much longer lasting and deeper reaching than 'happiness'.

The psychological, physical and emotional power of Decluttering

People generally love to surround themselves with stuff.

Clothes. Cooking equipment. Books (guilty!) Tools. Scrapbooking materials. Cameras. Knick knacks.

And much of this is worthwhile stuff. But not all. If you're anything like me, it's a delight to pick up a new article of clothing at the sales. And it makes perfect sense when you buy it, and then you get it home and find all the other clothes you have and wonder why you bought it in the first place.

Decluttering your wardrobe is a great way to get head space. The two don't sound connected, but if you are overwhelmed by choice every time you open the wardrobe door, then you could be seriously in the need of a clean out.

But which things to choose? You love them all, right?

Here's a great tip, that will see your own, shadow behaviour, make the decision for you, and I have to thank my friend Justin for this one.

Put all your coat hangers backwards. By that I mean have the hook facing the wardrobe opening. Every time you wear something, replace it on the clothes hanger in the normal way, that is, with the clothes hanger hook facing the back of the wardrobe.

Then, at the end of the season, have a look at all the clothes whose clothes hanger didn't change direction. You'll be self-selecting what you can get rid of without even realising it.

Obviously, this doesn't include formal wear or seldom worn items such as coats in warmer climates. But I think you get the idea.

This can be adapted to other things as well. Think of whatever your 'clutter' is, the clutter that you know deep down needs to be culled.

Then reverse something about it a la the coat hangers. Give yourself a reasonable time frame, and then let your own behaviour self-select what can stay, and what can go. It's very liberating.

You get the idea. Be ruthless, you'll be surprised at how much you really DON'T need. And if you are unsure, place the item/s in a plastic tub and pop it in the garage. If you haven't hunted for the item/s in 12 months, it's unlikely you'll ever need it again.

And you'll start feeling liberated from THINGS! Decluttering can just lighten your face up - it can literally be a weight coming off your shoulders - it almost makes you younger!

I have written a list of possible decluttering items. You might surprise yourself.

Here are some ideas for setting yourself free. You can make your clutter pay you (put it on Gumtree or eBay), or donating it can make a positive difference in someone else's life:

- Paperwork over seven years old
- Expired makeup
- Old, ugly underwear – life is too short
- Old technology such as leads, plugs, cables
- Clean out your medicine cabinet – check those due dates and ditch the old medications
- Clean out your pantry – again, check those due dates and ditch the out-of-date products
- Books you've finished with – a great charity option
- Jewellery you no longer wear
- Clothes that are more than two sizes too small. By the time you reach that goal, the fashions will have changed and you won't want to wear them anyway.
- Dust-collectors that no longer have any meaning for you (knick-knacks etc..)
- Old party supplies
- Old greeting cards – keep the sentimental ones, recycle the rest
- Used magazines – you could see if your local school wants them for kids' projects
- Rusty tools
- DVDs and CDs that are no longer to your taste
- Games, jigsaws, cards – anything you haven't used within the last 12 months
- Office supplies you haven't used in six months, including pens, white out, notebooks, filing systems etc...
- Kitchen utensils you have multiples of – such as cake tins, potato mashers, anything where just one will be enough
- Toys no longer cuddled
- Old keys
- Batteries that you don't know how long you've had
- Anything without a lid (eg plastic containers); any lids without a thing
- Travel brochures that are more than six months old
- Prescription glasses no longer used – most optometrists will take them off your hands and donate them to those who can't afford a new pair
- Remotes for electronics you no longer have or which no longer work

Beauty Sleep is not a myth

How do you sleep? Do you wake well-rested, or tired and grumpy? Do you need coffee to wake up?

What's your bedroom like? Do you have a TV in there? Maybe a digital clock. Do you keep your phone on your bedside table, charging, overnight? Do you keep your computer in your room?

Having these items in your bedroom can negatively impact your sleeping patterns. There are many studies from universities around the world that point to electromagnetic disturbance from electronics in the bedroom negatively impacting sleeping patterns.

There are also many studies about the colour of lights we are exposed to at night. Green and red lights (such as on your clock radio) are okay, but a blue light will upset your sleep patterns, so is a good one to stay away from.

If you have trouble sleeping, these guidelines may be worth following.

Always eat at least three hours before retiring. Avoid large meals in the evening, as your body will be focusing on digesting your food, rather than helping you relax enough to sleep. You could also suffer from indigestion, or worse, reflux, which can be painful, and life-threatening when combined with over-use of alcohol.

A couple of hours before you retire, start dimming the lights. Turn off the overhead lights and use side lighting, such as soft lamps. This will tell your body you are getting ready to retire for the night.

It's also worthwhile doing your teeth cleaning and skin cleansing routine a couple of hours before retiring - you don't want to be getting all nice and sleepy and then wake yourself up by turning on the bright bathroom light.

You might also try getting a small 'night' light to put in the toilet and/or bathroom so you don't have to turn on a light if you need a nighttime visit.

Use a lamp in the bedroom if you want to read. But DO NOT USE any technology, such as your phone, laptop, computer or tablet. Although these devices do provide us with many benefits, the downside of this technology is that the backlight of portable devices is blue - exactly the type of wavelength that disrupts sleep by delaying the production of melatonin.

Melatonin is needed to help you sleep. Interruption to that production impedes your ability to sleep well. So wait until morning to check your emails or Facebook. Don't worry, they will still be there.

Try to keep your bedroom cool and dark. The ideal is 18 degrees Celsius (about 65 degrees Fahrenheit).

Avoid alcohol before bedtime. Alcohol is a both a stimulant and a depressive, and too much of it affects the quality of your sleep. Other drinks to avoid include coffee, sports drinks, and anything else that is high in caffeine.

A nice way to get rest-ready is to have a bath (with lavender oil) Or you could lie on the floor with your legs up the wall. Believe it or not, it's very relaxing. Or this is where you could bring your nervous system under control by practicing that breathing technique I outlined earlier.

Finally, out of control stress can make it impossible for your mind to shut down. A good idea is to write down anything that's bothering you and leave it for the next morning. The actual process of writing can be a cue for your mind, and body, to let it go, even if it's just for a little while.

Reasons to enjoy being a sleepy-head and the benefit of naps

Your 'glial' cells (think of them like the housekeepers of your brain) come along at night and help build connections between your neurotransmitters such as dopamine and serotonin. 'Microglial cells' prune these connections. This research is pretty new, but it seems that the connections in your brain that you don't use often (maybe remembering names of people you've just met) get a protein attached to them (C1q). The microglial cell recognizes that C1q and destroys it. This is how, it is thought, your brain makes room for new information.

Have you ever wanted to release information from your brain out your ears? I remember starting a new job in IT once - and I had to go for walks in a nearby park twice a day because I was just feeling so overloaded with new information. Not just information - but a new IT language that bore absolutely no resemblance to anything I'd ever encountered.

This is a good example of how your brain works - and why you need a good night's sleep. Take my example of learning heaps in my new job. Although I did make a little bit of headway every day, my brain was just building temporary pathways, until it decided what I needed to remember, and what could be tossed out (think the C1q protein).

Obviously some of what I learned was important, and some I could get rid of. My brain did that - and used my sleep to carry out its search and destroy mission for the information that could be deleted. It also used this time to build stronger neural pathways for the information I needed to keep.

In fact, it's estimated that your brain cells shrink by about 60 percent at night to create space for the microglial cells to do their housekeeping job.

This is why, after a great night's sleep, you might feel you can think, and perhaps act, clearly and quickly.

Thinking with a brain that is deprived of sleep is like walking through treacle. It's sticky, bothersome and exhausting.

And napping? I'm a great napper. I can put my head down for 20 minutes and wake refreshed. My father spent many years as a journalist on the police rounds in the days before mobile phones - so what could you do when you were on a stakeout other than grab some shut-eye just in case you had to be awake for the next 20 hours. I think I got my ability to cat-nap from him.

So anyone who tells you napping is bad doesn't know what they're talking about (napping for over an hour is another matter - but that's not napping really is it, it's more like a sleep).

Sleep, cat nap and recharge. Give your lovely brain a chance to do its job - because it's doing it for you.

It's YOUR day, manage it YOUR way

It doesn't matter who you work for, whether it's yourself or someone else. It doesn't matter who your clients are. It doesn't matter if you live out of hotel rooms to go to work, or work at home. Your morning is yours, and, by setting it up right, you can own the rest of your day, regardless of your commitments and duties.

This is something I firmly believe. I now (as I have mentioned earlier) start my day with yoga practice, and then go to the gym. But this is not something I do because I work from home (or wherever I happen to be).

For many years (while working for others) I started my day by going for a morning walk before breakfast. It was my time for my head to clear, to think, to plan.

However, I had been making the mistake of starting my work day by opening my 'inbox' and using that to structure whatever was coming next. WRONG!!

I read something that made me rethink this completely. And I'd like to share it with you because I think it is so valuable, everyone should know it, and live by it.

'Spend 50 minutes in the morning stretching and strategising. Stretch for 20 minutes, then strategise your day for 30 minutes. This means you do not check email or respond to others in the first 50 minutes of the day. This alone will change your life.'

*'**The inbox is nothing but other people's agendas.** So if you begin the day in your inbox, you are framing the day in reaction, not thought. Instead, **get in tune with your body, then sit down and decide on the major projects and priorities** that you will dramatically move forward today.'*

- Brendon Burchard

BINGO! I can't tell you how much more in charge of my day I am now I don't open my inbox until midmorning. That may not be possible for everyone, but just give yourself that hour and a half (including breakfast!) and your life will change.

Taking time out and connecting with nature

The Japanese have a beautiful word for walking in the woods - Shinrin-yoku. It means 'forest bathing'. Isn't that lovely? Shinrin-yoku is known to boost immune function, reduce blood pressure and improve mood. But it's not just trotting through the forest, woods or bush blithely pushing on. You need to be 'mindful' - walk with your senses awakened so you absorb nature in a myriad of different ways.

Studies have shown that the microbes on the skin of people living close to vegetation (and a range of vegetation, not just oak trees, or coastal rosemary) are different - and these could directly affect immune function and mood.

So when you go walking in nature - really look at the leaves, the bark, the insects. Breathe deeply and fully and smell the different scents and aromas - not just the flowers, but the leaves, bark and grass. I mean, how wonderful does newly mowed grass smell. Touch nature (safely) and enjoy the different sensations on your skin. Enjoy these experiences as if you're doing them for the very first time. Get lost in nature - and you will find yourself.

Chapter 6
How do you make these changes stick?

'We are what we repeatedly do. Excellence, then, is not an act, but a habit.' - Aristotle

So the question now is - how do you start to make these changes?

I know people who hate structure. They say they don't like to be fenced in. I used to be like that. I wouldn't join a sports team or take up a weekly class because I might want to go away on a weekend and something would have to give - either my commitment or my trip away.

Then, of course, I had a job that made having a weekly anything impossible.

When I look back, I realise this attitude robbed me of something. I robbed myself of connections. I robbed myself of having a deeper experience of life.

Mostly I realised I had taken the idea of structure and made it a bad thing. I had made it something that had little or no value. So I turned it around and now I have structure in my life. This is structure that I choose, not structure that is imposed upon me.

That's the big difference of course. I am talking about something that I incorporate into my life to suit me, to benefit me, to serve me. Because now I realise what airlines have known forever - I am important. I am of value. I put on my own mask before helping others.

Routines are a form of structure. And implementing them can create great freedom.

Now I go to the gym five days a week. I don't think about it, I don't ask myself if I want to. I just do it. And I've started to love it.

I don't necessarily love the gym per se, not every day. But I do love knowing that I am doing something that will benefit me, that will help me stay strong, fit and healthy for the next phase of my life. It just means that the first thing I do in the day is for me.

I also have a routine where I care for my skin twice a day. I don't ask myself if I want to; I just do it. When I've finished brushing my teeth before retiring, I know the next steps are to cleanse, tone and moisturise my skin. It's a non-negotiable. I am never too tired to look after me. When I return from the gym I shower and cleanse, tone and moisturise, ready for the day.

Some interesting studies have been conducted on the importance of routine, and their value to us as humans.

Structure, or routine, can help provide direction in life. Without routine, you could well be rudderless. They provide a framework or guide to move life forward.

Routine helps efficiency - you will get far more done if you don't have to think about what's next - you can just do it.

Routine can relieve you of the burden of constant willpower, discipline and mental strain. As with my going to the gym in the morning, I don't have to have a 'will I, won't I' conversation with myself. I just do it.

Having a routine can help build momentum. If you want to shed kilos, for example, NOT having dessert may not seem like much, but build that up over 12 months and you will have made a big difference to your waistline.

It's similar with saving money. If you take your lunch to work rather than buying it, you might spend $50 a week less on food. Over a year you will have saved close to $2500 (this is assuming you work five days a week). I know a couple who lived frugally and took their lunch to work every day for eight years. That paid off their mortgage and they were in their early 30's when they owned their own home. Small steps can achieve big things.

You build competency. The more you do something, the better you get at it.

Rituals are also of great value to us as humans.

What's the difference between ritual and routine?

Well, routine is a consistent action or sequence of actions meant to achieve a particular outcome. Ritual has an emotional or even spiritual dimension attached to those actions. A Hen's night for a woman before she gets married is a ritual; so is Bar Mitzvah or Confirmation, Baptism or Christening. See the difference?

In a study conducted by the University of Minnesota, two groups were asked to eat chocolate, one following a precise ritual before consuming it, and the other group just eating it any old way. On average, the group who applied the ritual reportedly enjoyed the chocolate more, and thought it was a more expensive chocolate than those who just ate it without focus. They even tried the experiment on carrots and got similar results (not the value, just the taste).

So don't confuse Rituals and Routine. Just make them work for you.

Mind hacks to get new habits going

The three R's of habit formation

As much as 40 percent of our behaviour is habitual (Duke University). Researchers from Massachusetts Institute of

Technology (MIT) have termed this as a 'habit loop', and it consists of three components:

1. Cue or Trigger
2. Routine
3. Reward

(You might also hear it called the 3 R's - Reminder, Routine, Reward, which is what author Charles Duhigg has called the model).

The concept behind this model is that your behaviour is triggered by an event:

- Reminder or Cue: e.g. you come home exhausted after a long day.
- Routine: You throw down your laptop bag, handbag or briefcase on the lounge and reach for a glass of wine.
- Reward: you drink the wine and start to feel less stress.

If you view the Reward as a positive thing, e.g. the pressure reduces, and is replaced by a feeling of mellowness, then you'll repeat the pattern, and this reinforces the behaviour. Now this is great if you are doing something that is good for you - like exercising regularly.

But it's not so good if the behaviour, or habit, is detrimental to your health and wellbeing.

Here are brain hacks that might help with starting habits that will benefit you, or ditching habits that don't.

SMART goals

Some people swear by S.M.A.R.T goals. These goals are used in the corporate or business setting, but there is no reason why they can't be used to achieve personal goals.

- Specific - you need to be really clear what it is you want to achieve. For instance, is it weight loss, or getting healthier and stronger?

- Measurable - You won't achieve what you don't measure. If your aim is to be better at swimming, how will you know when you've achieved that? Is it successful stroke correction, or speed, or something else that will tell you that you are making progress.

- Attainable - you have to be realistic, which includes having a plan for when times get tough.

- Relevant - Is this goal the right thing at the right time for you to be focused on? Make sure it's going to complement your overall aims.

- Time-bound - be clear on when you want to achieve this by. This gives you an end point to focus on. And reward your efforts.

One Word

Another way to do it is to follow the *One Word* principle.

The One Word process is pretty simple. It was designed by Mike Ashcraft, pastor of a church in North Carolina, and he has since written a book with Rachel Olsen outlining its process. It consists of:

1. You think about who you want to be. Focus on the future, and think about the new you.

2. Make a list of the characteristics you want to see in the new you. You might think of someone you know who embodies these characteristics. Apply a one word description to each of these characteristics.

3. Once you have your list of one-word descriptions choose just one of those words that best articulates all that you want to be.

The idea is that one word is much easier to focus on. It's not something that you can get wrong, because it's what works for you.

Want to know my word? Well, lots came up for me but the one I settled on is......

focused.

The Motivation Wave

As I mentioned earlier, researchers have found that up to 40 percent of behaviours are accounted for by habits. When you think about it, it kind of explains why it's so hard to change a habit, or stop one.

We often say we 'lack motivation' or ' I just don't have the willpower'. But studies show that willpower is just like a muscle - sometimes it's strong, other times it's weak.

Stanford University professor BJ Fogg calls this the 'Motivation Wave'. It's not that you don't want to start a new habit, perhaps you're just choosing the wrong time of day, or you're trying to achieve too much change at once, or too many changes at once.

The Motivation Wave theory works like this. Say you want to exercise more. So rather than saying I'll go to the gym every day, start with just two or three visits a week. Start small, so that you build up the motivation muscle - rather than overloading it. The idea is that you...

'Make it so easy you can't say no.' - *Leo Babauta*

Small increases, big gains

Jim Rohn, master of motivation and clear thinking, had this to say about habits:

'Success is a few simple disciplines, practiced every day; while failure is simple a few errors in judgments, repeated every day.'

So just increasing what you want to do by, say, one percent per day, will see your habit improvements adding up really quickly.

Chunk it down

Chunking it down is a popular saying, but have you really thought about what it means?

Say you want to shed 10 kilos. That's a big number to start with, and could be a little bit scary. Start with a smaller goal - say two kilos by the end of next month. Then, when you've achieved that goal, you set the next one - two kilos in six weeks. (Just so there's no confusion, I'm not recommending that specific loss in that time frame, it's simply a Chunking Down illustration.)

Getting back on track

Neuroscientist Kelly McGonigal suggests, *'The best way to improve your self-control is to see how and why you lose control'*. What are the triggers for you? In what environment do you exhibit the behaviour?

Rather than being an all-or-nothing type - know that you will drop the ball sometimes when you're trying to install a new habit.

Because you know that, you can plan for those times. Want to go Dry July (that is, not drink alcohol for the month of July)? And then a work function comes up that you have to go to? Prepare for that. Have a plan to help you through it. Are there daily issues that challenge your desire for change?

We all fail sometimes. Successful people have strategies for this:

1. They have plans for when they fail. They know the triggers or dangers and prepare for them.

2. They get back on track very quickly.

3. They forgive themselves when they drop the ball.

Consistency here is the most important thing. As my mate Nick Cownie says, **progress, not perfection,** is key.

Implementation Intention

Psychology Professor Peter Gollwitzer has found that if people write down **exactly** what they are going to do, and where they are going to do it, they will be more successful in actually doing it.

Let's take meditation as an example. The Implementation Intention works simply by reframing your goals into IF statements, and the IF becomes a cue for the action to take place:

'IF I'm in bed at night, I'll meditate for five minutes before I pick up my book/crossword.'

Perhaps it's a bad habit, say losing your temper. It could work like this:

'IF I find my blood starting to boil, I'll take three deep breaths before I speak.'

Habit Stacking

Habit stacking works a little differently. This is a pretty simple technique, which requires you to stack one new habit onto an existing one.

For instance:
- 'Before taking my shower, I'll do a five minute Salute to the Sun stretch.'
- 'After I get into bed, I'll write in my journal.'

To start using this strategy, write two lists:

1. The habits you already have (you'll be surprised how many of them there are) and

2. The ones you wish to start (don't go overboard now).

Now pair up the new habits you want to start, with a natural fit (as in the example above). Start with just one or two, and build up over time.

Patience and pacing

Patience is probably the hardest thing to master. I know it's not one of my strengths and I need to practice it every day. When trying to make a change, pick a strategy you're pretty sure you can sustain.

Let's take exercising again. There are many ways you could do exercise. Going to the gym is one of them.

But this may not work for you because:
- it's too far away,
- you can't get there as often as you would like, or
- you just don't like the gym.

So do something else. Sign up for a yoga class, or check the MeetUps in your area and see if there is a walking group. See what a colleague or friend would like to do and buddy up - sometimes having a commitment to someone else makes it easier to keep your commitment to yourself.

Find something you want to try, and commit eight weeks to it. At the end of that time, you'll know if it's something you can sustain and be consistent about. Then you can add something else to your exercise regime.

It doesn't matter what you do as much as it matters that you do it, consistently. This will get you the long term achievements you are looking for.

Commitment Contract

As human beings, we don't like to lose. Or to be seen to back out of a commitment.

A Commitment Contract is a way to harness our humanness into a strategy that can be highly motivating. It's easy to hit that snooze button, or sneak in a chocolate bar when no-one is watching. But what if someone were….?

A Commitment Contract helps keep you honest.

1. Write down your goal e.g. do a five minute Salute to the Sun stretch every morning.

2. Have something at stake. Like cash, or your reputation.

3. Have a referee - a friend or a coach who will hold you accountable.

Place your goal where you will see it every day. Share your goal with your friend or coach, agree on a way for you to keep them posted about your progress. For instance, you have to take a selfie while doing your stretch routine and share it with your coach. If you don't, you have to pay a charity $20, or post your failure to do it on social media.

Surfing the Urge - dealing with bad habits

Other research has identified a way to help break habits. It's called 'Surfing the Urge'.

Let's say you work long and hard (no great stretch of the imagination because I know you do). You finally stagger home after an 11 hour day, throw down the laptop and handbag, and reach for a *fill-in-the-blank* (eg a glass of wine).

Some neuroscientists believe that we do this because when that urge comes up, we are driven to feeding it as we think that will make it go away. But in fact, it doesn't. It makes the urge stronger.

The Surfing the Urge approach is simple - acknowledge the urge, sit with it. Say 'Yes, I would like a glass of wine', then pour yourself a glass of water, and just sit with the urge. Scientists are discovering the urge really does go away of its own accord when it's not fed.

*   *   *   *   *

There are many theories about forming new habits, and breaking bad ones. It may take a while for you to identify which is the best one for you.

But the important thing is you keep going. And forgive yourself for when you slip up.

A number of studies have been conducted looking at how we treat ourselves when we do slip up. The results are very interesting. Most people tend to harshly criticize themselves when they drop the ball. I bet you do. I can almost hear it. 'Idiot!' 'Oh you putz' (this is my husband's favourite). Or 'That's right dumbass, you've screwed up again.'

This is SO counter-productive. Research shows that this kind of self-criticism only makes you feel worse, and reduces your ability to meet your goals.

Successful people have a different approach. They reframe their setbacks as information, data, that they can use. They know that setbacks are unavoidable, so they don't sweat them. Instead they use them to learn.

Instead of 'You idiot, you know you like a cigarette after pizza - so why the hell did you eat pizza!' a successful person might say: 'Ah, I've had my pizza and now I could really do with a cigarette. That's good to know - next week I'll have the Lemon Veal'. (And maybe they feel like a cigarette after Lemon Veal. So the next week they might think, 'Hmm, maybe I should try Thai'.)

These are very top level ideas to show you there are many ways to start, stop and change habits. I hope the research I've provided here gives you some useful starting points. It may take you a while to find the strategy that is right for you. Your first attempt may not work as well as you might like it to when you are starting off. So remember, be kind to yourself.

If you criticise yourself, you'll just set your journey back. Start to study yourself, your behaviours, and particularly your self-talk, because the best thing you can do is learn about yourself.

Ways to say NO

And just one more thing, as promised in Chapter 3. Saying NO is absolutely VITAL to your peace of mind, and your time. If you can't say no, then you'll need to learn. And leave the word sorry out.

The idea here is to be strong, and firm, and sound like you would if you were advising a dear friend not to take on too much. You can always make a suggestion about how the person asking might get their request answered. You might even get the reputation as the 'go-to' girl for suggestions, which frees up loads of time.

No.   No thanks, I won't be able to make it.

Not this time.   No thanks, I have another commitment.

Maybe another time.   I'm booked into something else.

Thanks, but no thanks.   I've got too much on my plate right now.

I'm not taking on anything else right now.

Bandwidth is low, so I won't be able to make it work.

If only I could!   I'd love to — but can't.

Darn! Not able to fit it in.   I'm slammed.

Perhaps next season when things clear up.

Thanks for thinking of me, but I can't help you this time.

I'm not the girl for you on this one.

I'm learning to limit my commitments.

Another time might work, but not today.

It doesn't sound like the right fit for me.

My word of the year is REST, so I can't fit another thing in.

I'm not the best fit for it. Maybe you could try xxx

No thank you, it sounds lovely but I'm not able to help/attend/
join in.

It sounds like you're looking for something I'm not able to give
right now.

Not now.   If only I had a clone!

I won't be able to dedicate the time needed to do a good job.

I'm immersed in something big right now so won't be able to help.

I wish there were two of me!   I'm honoured, but can't.

**Because being kind to yourself
is really the whole point of this book.**

Chapter 7

This all sounds great, but where do you find the time?

'All the flowers of all of the tomorrows are in the seeds of today.' – Chinese Proverb

And isn't that the thing? You are super-busy, and I hope that I have made it clear that I really, really understand that.

Children. Husband. Partner. Siblings. Parents. Extended family. Work. Committees. Clubs. Everyone wants a piece of you. And if you want to do just half of what I talk about in this book, where on earth will you find the time? And you know you want to, because, like that well-known advertisement says, you are worth it.

So I have two things to say about that.

1. Get rid of the idea of perfection.
2. Learn to enjoy outsourcing.

Focusing on perfection is really focusing on imperfection.

Seriously. If you are just wanting everything to be perfect, how often do you find it so? And when you don't, what do you find? Imperfection. The kitchen bench with crumbs. The dishes in the sink. Your kids' clothes on the bedroom floor. Your husband's/ partner's clothes on the bedroom floor! Dust bunnies under the bed. Streaks of toothpaste on the bathroom sink. Hair in the shower. The bin needing emptying. The ironing done. The lunches made.

These are all real, important things. But they don't have to be done to perfection. You will be continually disappointed if your standards are so high that you are never satisfied. Not only does perfection limit your enjoyment of life, it could make you hard to live with.

I know some women for whom perfection is a daily goal. They are terminally striving to achieve that which is unachievable, especially when so much of that requires the cooperation of others.

Children generally aren't neat. They won't do things the way you want them too. But if they help (or have household tasks to do - which frankly I think every child should) then as long as they have done it to the best of their ability - isn't that enough? Sure, they could learn to do something better - and will do as they mature. And your job, partly, is to teach them. But it doesn't have to be all at once, does it?

And if you don't have kids, but have an errant partner - well. Perhaps you could compromise a bit more? Perhaps the dishwasher doesn't really need to be stacked the *exact* way you prefer. Or the clothes don't need to be hung out according to your rules? Or the sheets folded exactly along the lines.

I know, these things can make life easier. If the sheets are hung 'properly', it makes it easier to know where the middle is to make the bed. But will it stop you from sleeping well? Isn't that more important?

Or if the dishwasher needs a load to be put on a few plates earlier than if you'd packed it - well, not much will ride on it, really.

If you are a perfectionist - what are your hot buttons? What are the things that you really feel can't be done in any other way than the way you do them?

Perhaps you could sit down and write a list. You partner and/or family could help (without being sarcastic).

Then perhaps you could really look at that list and identify where you could compromise.

Because when you compromise on these items, two things will happen. You can let go of responsibility for everything in the world. And your mind will start to clear. You will have room for other things. What other things? YOU.

And if that can't happen, then…..

Outsource

Yes. Pay someone else to do these things for you.

This may take a bit more of an effort, particularly if you are looking to have a longer term arrangement. But it will be worth it.

Just imagine, you wake up on a Saturday morning, and
- you won't have to clean the house
- you won't need to do the washing
- you won't need to have the car washed / serviced.

But what other things can you outsource? How about:
- Housekeeping.
- Shopping.
- Cleaning.
- Ironing.
- Putting together the new flatpack furniture.
- Taxes.
- Administrative bits and pieces.
- Scrubbing the tiles.
- Spring clean.
- Mowing.
- Gardening.
- Looking after the pool.
- Putting out the garbage.

- Cooking meals.
- House repairs.
- Small plumbing jobs.
- Sweeping the patio.
- Driving.
- Collection of items such as drycleaning or parcels.
- Computer issues.
- TV, stereo or other technical stuff.
- Drive your car around the block while you're on holidays.
- Take photos of a birthday party.
- Design the invitations to a farewell party.
- Research a gift.
- Research for an overseas trip.
- Selling a car.

You really can outsource pretty much anything these days. Tim Ferris, author of the '*4 Hour Work Week*', even outsourced his dating. If you need it, you can outsource it.

You can place an ad in Gumtree.com. You could checkout Airtasker. com, upwork.com, or fiverr.com. Ask friends who they use. Give yourself some time back - it's the only thing in this world you can't make more of.

Chapter 8
Your skin - it's a wrap!

'Love yourself first and everything else will fall into line. You really have to love yourself to get anything done in this world.' - Lucille Ball

I hope you have enjoyed my book, and have learned something too.

I have wanted to just share - not preach. This whole book is driven out of my own experience. Working in corporate Australia was a real privilege, but came at a cost too. Some people were terrifically supportive, others backstabbing. And if you work in the corporate world, or run your own business - you might experience the same thing. Rather than looking after myself - I often did things that didn't serve me. I took a path that saw great achievements - but also great suffering - with my health, my emotions and my spirituality.

And I want your way to be different to mine. I want you to be kind to yourself.

A brief recap might be called for here. Because although it's a skinny book - I have covered quite a bit of stuff!

There's no getting around it - what you put into your body will show on your face and in the quality of your skin. And nowhere is this more important than how you treat your gut.

Supporting your digestive system is essential for your health - short and long term. Without a healthy gut, your immune system will suffer.

I mean, just because it's winter - why should we all get a cold or the flu? I know that travelling regularly on aircraft or public transport might put you right in the thick of it. Working in air-conditioned buildings might also leave you at risk. But some people suffer from multiple colds or 'flu in a season. And they might get other illnesses that require antibiotics - which, although wonderful and I wouldn't be without them - act as napalm for all gut flora - not just the nasties. It might be a different story if your immune system was better supported.

There are a number of ways you can support your gut health. Fibre (keeping things moving), prebiotics and probiotics are essential. Good oral health will help keep bacteria at bay. In fact, I know I didn't cover oral health much, but a healthy mouth can make a huge difference to your overall health. Whatever is in your mouth will find its way into the rest of your body - think how absorbent your skin is, as well as bacteria flowing down your intestinal tract with food. So please make sure you visit your dentist regularly, and look after your mouth - teeth, gums and tongue.

Focusing on what and how you eat can also help. Chewing your food really well is essential to reduce the pressure on your digestive system, and to get the most nutrient benefit from your food. Eating in a calm state (not in front of the TV or computer) can also help. If you are rushing to get that report done while shoving a sandwich down your throat, you will really not be focused will you?

Drinking lots of water is also helpful to keep yourself hydrated. Studies have shown that often we mistake hunger for thirst - so 250ml eight times per day will really help you. And it's not just your gut - staying hydrated will also help your skin to stay smooth and put off the wrinkles - isn't that reason alone to drink water?

Speaking of wrinkling - it is a sad fact that our skin loses elasticity as we get older. Our skin is truly magical and does many things for us such as keeping the bad stuff out, and keeping the good stuff in (like our insides).

The important thing to remember is that, while you can't stop your skin from ageing, you can slow it down by looking after it. You are surrounded by things that are bad for your skin - pollution, excess coffee and alcohol, over exposure to the sun, stress, poor sleep, making sub-optimal food choices are just a few. You may not be able to stop your wrinkles, but you can slow them down with loving care of yourself.

Which brings me to a regular beauty routine. Not just because looking after your skin is worth your time. But also because looking after **YOU** is worth your time.

Who else will look after you if you won't? Who will be a good role model for your children if you won't?

Having a regular routine is good for you. It is self care, self nourishment, self nurture. When we do these things for others, we, as women, are praised. We know inside ourselves they are valuable activities (that's why we do them) - so why don't we do them for ourselves? It doesn't take much time - just checking out my skin routine videos shows how little time it would take out of your day.

So what's stopping you? Don't give me that 'no time, too busy' baloney. You have time to look after others, children, partners, parents, colleagues. It's time you carved out just a little bit for yourself. And I truly believe those who love you will support you in this.

Having a regular routine for looking after your skin is not just a superficial act.

There is a lot of research that shows our cells - the building blocks of life - react well to positive vibrations. And if that's too much esoteric stuff for you, just take a look at Dr Emoto's work with water crystals.

Our cells, the building blocks of life, are like water crystals, and react to the vibrations around them. Looking after yourself, even just for 10-15 minutes a day (that's only five minutes in the morning if you think about it), will communicate itself to your body.

The few minutes a day can also include your food choices. When you're out and about, it's really easy to fall into to the trap of grabbing the easiest thing to eat. If you're doing what I used to do and traveling for work, then going out to dinner or buying pre-prepared meals can be about all you can manage. But there are better ways to care for yourself.

Protein shakes are a good option - especially if you're going to eat late. Recent research shows that it's not just what you eat, but when you eat is also crucial. If you feel you are carrying too much fat, and/or if you sleep poorly, your eating habits could be part of the problem. A late night meeting, meaning a late dinner, can be doubly bad for you. It's best for you to try to leave two to three hours between your last meal and retiring. And if that's impossible, then perhaps something light like a protein shake and a small share of almonds or walnuts before the meeting would serve you better.

When you do have time to cook at home, whole foods - those with the least amount of human intervention - are really best.

There are many ways you can cook well, and quickly.

In summer, salads, smoothies, juices, stir fries are just a few ideas. In winter, my favourite is a slow cook something, or a piece of poached fish with steamed vegetables and a lemon sauce. Easy to make, super easy to eat.

I really don't believe it's easier to eat badly - it's all about food choices and priorities. I know a woman who never cooked for herself. In fact, she lived in a small apartment for three months before discovering it had no oven. She lived on TV dinners and packaged foods. Her skin looked terrible, and after many years of following this diet, she was diagnosed with Insulin-dependent Type 2 diabetes. Type 2 diabetes can also leave you vulnerable to heart disease (currently the biggest killer of women in Australia and New Zealand, with stroke being the second biggest killer).

These killers are lifestyle diseases - and preventable. My grandmother had a stroke at 82, and I spent the next four years watching her die. It was awful and I wouldn't wish that on anyone. I certainly don't want YOU experiencing it because you opted for the easy choices rather than caring about yourself.

Even if you do eat whole foods, take time over your meals. Be kind to your digestion.

It's very easy to make choices with canned and packaged goods that don't serve you. (Food manufactures are getting super-sneaky - particularly with labeling and hiding sugar.) So please, check your pantry and ditch all those items that have high levels of sugar, salt, and can't claim a BPA free can lining.

It's the little things that can add up, and that can show up in your waistline, and your skin and health further down the track.

This of course, brings me to supplementing your diet. As you know, I'm a believer in taking quality supplements. All the organic food in the world can't deliver you the vitamins and minerals that don't exist in the soil to start with.

Our modern farming practices have really had a huge impact on the quality of our foods. So do yourself a favour - have a look at my website (www.enrichyourenergy.usana.com) and do some research. Go to YouTube, and do some research. Go to Google, and do some research. You are worth it. And if you want to chat - I'm here (meredith@meredithyardley.com).

MY NUTRITION

EMAIL ME

Once you've had a good sleep, eaten a good meal, there's one thing left of course. Exercise. Movement. Being flexible. Doesn't matter what you do, just do it. Walk. Swim. Yoga. Dance. Tai Chi.

There's a guy at my gym who arrives in a wheel chair. His disability doesn't stop him working out. When I lived in Sydney I used to see a guy riding a bike. Now that might not sound very unusual - but he only had one leg. That's inspiring.

There is no excuse not to do something. Just figure out what movement you love to do, and make it fit in to your life. As Dr. Levine says, '*we are sitting ourselves to death*'. Please choose living with joy - and MOVE.

* * * *

If communicating self-compassion to your body is so positive at a cellular level, think what it also does to your mindset.

There are many things you can do regularly (every day or so) that will make yourself feel fabulous.

- Breathe mindfully
- Set a daily intention
- Meditate / Reflect
- Be thankful / grateful
- Declutter (this may be more like a once a year thing)
- Sleep well and refreshingly - which includes getting rid of the electronics that can disturb your sleep patterns.

95

Remember to have fun

Most importantly (to my mind) is to get your good habits installed, and give the bad ones the heave-ho. There are many ways you can do this.

Maybe the SMART goal strategy would work for you.

Or perhaps the One Word strategy is more appealing.

Surfing the Urge to get rid of the bad habits is a great start. You could journal how you're feeling, or you could identify trigger events and avoid them. These are both good ways to take control of the bad habits.

Patience and Pacing, Habit Stacking and Commitment Contracts are also good approaches.

It seems to me that there are few themes in the approaches I've outlined:

- Be specific - say 'I will to eat four servings of veggies a day' rather than just 'I want to eat healthy'.

- Get support - buddy up with someone or ask for their help. This could be as simple as wanting to get healthier, so ask a friend to go walking with you three days a week.

- Prepare for challenges - you know things will get in the way when you want to establish something new. Think of what these challenges might be, and have a plan to deal with them in advance. That way obstacles won't derail you.

- Be flexible - following on from the point above, if something really gets in the way, then go with the flow, be gentle with yourself and others, and re-plan. You will be more successful in the long run than if you're rigid about it. Consistency is key. And so is self-compassion.

All I really want for you is to take the steps, make the changes, slowly is fine - that will serve you. That will see you be a happier, healthier, more fulfilled you.

Please let me know how you go. I'd love to hear about your successes!

Resources

Because I want you to get stuck straight into looking after yourself, I have listed a bunch of resources I use. These are not just ideas or things someone else has suggested, I have truly used each and every one of them, so I offer them from my positive experience:

Outsourcing and Time Management:

- Success Automation: A big recommendation for me is an investment of three days at a course in Sydney, Australia, called Success Automation. I love all the courses that Authentic Education runs, and this one is a doozy. (They also have lots of great trainings you can buy to help you be the best you can be. Check it out here.)

AUTHENTIC EDUCATION

- gumtree.com. Great for regional and rural areas (in Australia is my experience), you can find anyone to do anything - a one-off cleaning job or a regular lawn mowing and pool scrubbing service. Ironing, typing - you name it, just place an ad and someone will answer. I even recently saw an ad from a single, hard working man who just wanted someone to cook him really good quality meals so he didn't have to live on take-away. And he hasn't even read my book!

- airtasker.com. Terrific if you live in the city, you can get people to do anything. Put your flat pack furniture together or set up your media entertainment system. It's worth a look for two reasons - you'll be freeing up your own time, and helping someone else.

- <u>Evernote</u>. An app that acts like your electronic brain (complete with an elephant logo - there's the hint). There are only three things you need to do, remember to download it, remember to write your messages in it (eg shopping list, things to talk to the doctor about), and remember to look in it. It's a brilliant device and I'd be lost without it.

- <u>Upwork</u>. I have used the services here to edit this book, as well as some digital marketing work, but the list here is really endless: administration, web design, marketing, customer service, writing, translation, even analytics and engineering. You could even use this for researching that special gift, designing birthday invitations, or preparing that school fete poster.

- <u>Fiverr.</u> Outsource that graphic design, programming, video or animation work. If you haven't signed a non-disclosure agreement with your employer or client, you may even use Upwork or Fiverr for business, and you certainly can if you run your own business.

Other Resources to care for yourself

- <u>Free Health Assessment</u>: if you are really serious about your health, then get a great start by finding out where your health level sits with this free assessment. You will be given a confidential report and recommendations and suggestions about changes you can consider making to be the best 'you' that you can possibly be. (www.enrichyourenergy.usana.com)

FREE HEALTH ASSESSMENT

- Yoga apps: Daily Yoga and Yoga Studio. I use both depending on my mood.

- Fitbit - which also requires purchasing the flex or whichever model you choose. Great for keeping on track with movement, calorie intake and expenditure, and water counting. You really can't achieve what you don't measure.

- Words with Friends app. I have to admit, I'm an addict. It's a great stress relief and keeps my brain moving, without being too demanding. There's a free version with ads, and a paid version without. And I get to keep up to date with existing overseas friends, and make some new ones.

- DarrenDaily@darrenhardy.com. Darren Hardy is an American author, keynote speaker, advisor and a bunch of other things, but what I love about him is his little two minute podcasts every morning. Gets me set up just right.

- Easy Stool. (Australia) This will absolutely help you with good poop posture.

- Go outside. Enjoy the sun, grass, fresh air, trees, plants, beach, sand, woodland creatures. Just get outside and chill.

Quality Nutritional Supplements Checklist

Here is my checklist that I use to make sure that my **nutritional supplements** meet a number of criteria:

- They must be potency guaranteed, which means that what it says on the bottle must be in the product.

- They must be manufactured by the company selling them. The manufacturing processes must be rigorous, with a guarantee of no contamination. For instance, I want to be absolutely certain there is no mercury in my fish oil supplements.

- The manufacturer must open themselves up to external auditing by well-regarded groups (such as the American Independent Public Health and Safety Organization NSF International, and The Therapeutic Drugs Administration in Australia).

- The manufacturing process must be to pharmaceutical standards, not food standards which is what most nutritional supplements companies are made to. Pharmaceutical standards are those by which our drugs are made, whether non-prescription or prescription. It simply raises the quality bar much higher.

- I want to be certain of the bioavailability of the supplements I take. That means I want the goodness getting into my system as soon as possible.

- I want to know that everything on the label is in the product, so all the better if elite and Olympic athletes use them too. I know they have too much at stake to risk taking something that isn't reliable, or that can leave them exposed to disqualification due to accidently absorbing banned substances.

- And I like the companies I deal with to have a robust ecological mindset, to walk gently on this planet.

Skin Care Product Checklist

To check out the skin care I usego to my website: www. enrichyourenergy.usana.com - you can even order product for yourself! (You can email me if you have any problems).

ORDERING

EMAIL FOR PROBLEMS

My guiding principles are:

- Always buy the best quality you can afford.

- Choose products that have a botanical base.

- Use a day moisturiser that has at least an SPF factor 15. If you want more coverage try a mineral foundation.

- Choose products that are dripping with good quality vitamins and other minerals to nourish your skin's cells. Good starting points are:
   - Vitamin C assists collagen production and improves skin tone and smoothness.
   - Vitamin A helps with healing and creating new skin tissue.
   - Vitamin E is an antioxidant which helps protect against free radical damage.
   - Zinc helps repair and strengthen tissue.

- Grapeseed extract is a highly potent antioxidant to protect the skin.
- Beta carotene helps maintain the integrity of all cell membranes and your digestive system.
- Omega 3s help feed the cells, keeping them plump.

- Choose products that have independent scientific evidence behind them, proving they do what they say they do. Ask to see the results and if they can't show the results, then really why would you use the product.

- Choose products that have no chemical nasties (email me for my bonus chapter on this). That includes looking for BHP-free packaging.

- Choose products that have packaging that protects the product - i.e. that you don't stick your finger or applicator in. This will ensure no bacteria enters the product.

- Check that the packaging is treated so it can't leak into your product, and visa versa.

- Choose a product provider that make the products themselves, not one who engages a third party to make it and then just slaps their label on it. That way you can be sure that what is on the ingredients list is actually in the product.

Questions for you to think about when choosing personal care products:

- What preservation system do they use?

- If they don't use a preservative, how is the product protected from moulds, fungus and bacteria?

- What is the shelf life? Do you need to refrigerate it?

- In what sort of facility are these products produced? If it's a lady with a stall down at the markets with a homemade product, I can assure you that she is not preparing these in a clinically clean environment, no matter how earnest she is about their 'natural' or 'organic' ingredients.

- If the name on the label is not the name of the manufacturer, how do they ensure the manufacturing process is rigorous? What else do they make in the factory and what steps are taken against cross contamination?

- What sort of packaging do they use? If it's plastic, is it BPA free? (If you've been living in a cave, BPA is Bisphenol A. A limited amount of research has shown that BPA can seep into food or beverages from containers that are made, or lined, with BPA. The concerns about BPA exposure include possible health effects on the brain, behaviour and prostate glands of foetuses, infants and children.)

- How do they ensure the product doesn't leach into the packaging, and vice versa? If it's glass, do they line the inside of the glass with anything?

- What sort of testing do they do? Do they test on animals? (This may not be important to you, but it is essential for some people to know that animals were not harmed in the preparation of the products they use. I am one of them.)

- Do they open themselves up to external independent auditing such as the American NSI?

- What clinical studies do they have to support their product does what they say it does?

- Are the products you use made to work with each other? If not, how can you be sure they won't work against each other?

- What does the exfoliator use as its roughage? Is it small plastic balls? You'd be surprised how many exfoliators contain this (and as recently as August 2015, California has banned them in products because of the huge environmental - particularly marine - damage they do).

- What sort of research and development goes into the product?

- Do they have a screw-top lid with a wide opening? Do you stick your finger in the product? If you do, you're contaminating your product from the get-go.

References
(I did LOTS of reading so you don't have to.)

- Brendon Burchard, *The Motivation Manifesto,* 2014, Hay House Inc, USA
- Catherine Auman, LMFT, *Shortcuts to Mindfulness*, 2014, Green Tara Press, Los Angeles, USA
- Chris Crowley & Henry S. Lodge, MD, *Younger Next Year*, 2007, Workman Publishing Company Inc, New York, USA
- David Heller, ND, www.doctoroz.com, 30 July 2012, USA
- Dr Karl Kruszelnicki, *Brain Food*, 2011, Pan Macmillan Australia Pty Ltd, Australia
- Dr Monica Lewis & Dr Gerald Lewis, Dietary Supplements, 2007, MixMedia, New Zealand
- Dr. Phillippe Grandjean and Philip J. Landrigan, MD, *The Lancet*, Volume 13, Issue 3, in March 2014 edition, United Kingdom
- Dr Regina Hamlin, Dr Peter McDonald, Glenn Putnam, *The Science of Sensé*, Usana Health Sciences, Utah, USA
- Dr Sarah McKay, *Neuroscience Insight, How to Break Bad Habits*, Chopra Centre, Jan 2016, www.chopra.com
- European Commission on Endocrine Disruption (ECED), http://ec.europa.eu/environment/chemicals/endocrine/index_en.htm
- Giulia Enders, *Gut - The Inside story of our body's most under-rated organ*, Scribe Publications, 2015, Brunswick, Victoria, Australia (Translated from the original German *Darm Mit Charme*, Ullstein, 2014).
- Guy Croton (producer), *100 Best Ways to Stay Young*, 2011, Parragon, United Kingdom
- *Harvard Health Publications*, Harvard University, September 2015, USA
- *Health & Fitness Magazine*, Volume 21, 2014, Blitz Publications, Australia
- James Clear, http://jamesclear.com/habit-guide
- Jane Campsie, *face, Marie Claire style*, 2007, Murdoch Books, Australia
- Kenton, Leslie & Kenton, Sussanah, *The Authentic Woman*, 2005, Vermilion, United Kingdom

- Lyle MacWilliam MSc, FP, *Comparative Guide to Nutritional Supplements*, 2013, Northern Dimensions Publishing, USA
- Mayo Clinic, *www.mayoclinic.org*, September 2015, USA
- *MedicalNewsToday.com*, September 2015, USA
- Medical Research Education, www.mreassociates.org. references Fairfield KM, Fletcher RH, 2002
- National Geographic, *Your Body: A User's Guide*, 2014, National Geographic Society, USA
- National Geographic, *Your Personality Explained*, 2014, National Geographic Society, USA
- Readers' Digest, *Looking after your body*, 2003, Readers' Digest (Australia) Pty Ltd, Australia
- S.J. Scott, *Habit Stacking*, CreateSpace publishing, 2014
- *Sodium Laurel Sulphates: The Facts,* SLS free.net, 2016
- United States Department of Agriculture, www.ams.usda.gov, October 2012, USA
- US National Library of Medicine, May 2014, https://www.nlm.nih.gov, USA
- Victorian Government, Australia, www.betterhealth.vic.gov.au, August 2014
- Wiley Online Library, *Influence of Body Position on Defecation in Humans*, 2010, http://onlinelibrary.wiley.com/doi/10.1111/j.1757-5672.2009.00057.x/abstract

About the author

Meredith spent many years working for some of Australia's largest institutions in the corporate world in media, public relations, communication and change management. After unexpectedly, but delightfully, finding her life partner in 2010, Meredith became a self-confessed 'corporate refugee' - turning her back on the corporate world.

A lifelong interest in health and wellbeing led her to bring her experience in communication and change management to a broader audience - those wishing to make changes to their health and lifestyle, but not quite sure how to do it, where to start or how to make it stick.

'Helping busy women have abundant health and wealth' has become Meredith's passion. Because she has led that busy life, long hours at the office, high pressure and occasionally hostile work environments, living in hotel rooms and out of suitcases, and driving herself until her health suffered, she wanted to share her experiences with others so they can make the changes necessary so they don't have to feel old, poor and sick.

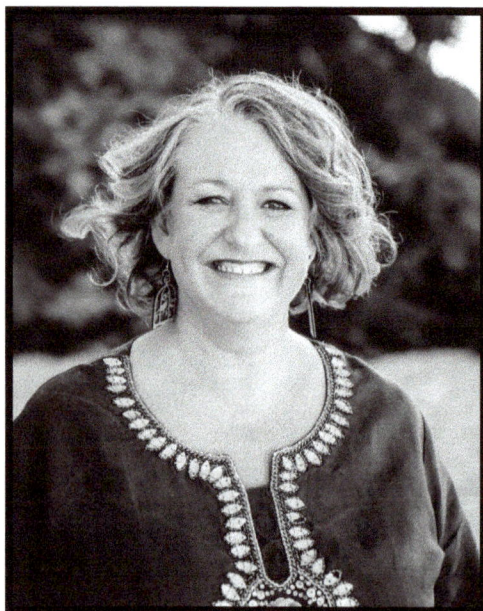

Abundant health and wealth - if you want it, connect with Meredith now.

Email: meredith@meredithyardley.com

Website: www.meredithyardley.com

Facebook: www.facebook.com/enrichingyourenergy

What Busy Women from around the world have said about the
Busy Woman's Guide to Inner Health and Outer Beauty

Here's what some busy women from our global village had to say about Meredith's book. These women work in business, music, health, financial services - yet their message is remarkably similar:

'I read '*The Busy Woman's Guide to Inner Health and Outer Beauty*' and just couldn't put it down. Meredith's research is truly impressive and I thought I knew a thing or two about the health of the skin and body. This book goes deep into not only the physical aspect of healthy inner and outer vibrance but the spiritual and emotional as well. The busy woman who says she has no time for herself should do herself a favour and make this compulsory reading. Loved it.'
Anne Noonan, Yoga and Wellness Lifestyle Coach, Brisbane, Australia, www.annenoonan.com.au

'I'm so excited about EVERYTHING Meredith has shared in this book. It's my new bible! So nice and refreshing to read and so easy to understand. It's not hard nor does not really take up time, but it's important to adapt to a healthy life for both inner health and outer beauty....'
Danielle Virgona, busy full-time working mum of a toddler, Hong Kong

'Wow thank you so much for sending me your fabulous book to review! I love the easy, chatty style of writing, great information and practical tips! Even as an experienced Wellness Coach and Nutrition Adviser this book enriched my knowledge and I am certain that everyone who reads it will gain many ah-ha moments and little gems to enhance their life!'
Dee Constable, busy mum and grandmum, Wellness Coach and Nutrition Adviser, Perth, Australia www.deeconstable.com.au

'I found this reading to be a concise, insightful, and inspiring compilation of techniques and positive daily practices, all here, all researched, and all in one place. Like a daily "how to" guide to live longer and feel and look younger! I am excited to set some goals and make some positive changes in my life and daily routines.'
Susan Purton, busy full-time working mum of three teenagers, Vancouver, Canada

'I got lots of useful information from it! Some of it was new stuff, some was confirmation of things I already knew and/or suspected. It was all clear and direct - EXACTLY what we busy women need!! No guilt trips, no excess guff, and options for different schedule and lifestyle choices. In short I LOVED IT!!'
Rachel Taylor, busy working singer, songwriter, musician, London, UK

'As a mother of two and about to turn 40 next year it was a great way to be given a wake up call about health. Great tips on how to improve all aspects of yourself - physically and mentally.'
Gloria Williams, busy full-time working mother of two toddlers, Brisbane, Australia

With thanks

My beloved husband, Henri, without whose unfailing love, support and belief I would never have finished this book.

My mum, Maggie, who has inspired me to achieve throughout my life.

Professional Endurance Triathlete, Michelle Duffield, who found time in her super-busy schedule to pen my Foreword.

www.ingramcontent.com/pod-product-compliance
Lightning Source LLC
Chambersburg PA
CBHW052012030426
42334CB00029BA/3196